I0024824

MYSTERIES OF THE MIND
Two Astonishing Articles that Solve the Mystery

MICHAEL R. BINDER, M.D.

The University of Chicago
Pritzker School of Medicine

MYSTERIES OF THE MIND:
Two Astonishing Articles that Solve the Mystery

© Copyright 2021 Michael R. Binder, M.D.
All Rights Reserved.

ISBN: 978-0-9748836-7-0

TABLE OF CONTENTS

Rethinking the Mind-Brain Duality:
Converging Lines of Evidence Shed New Light on the Anatomy
of Consciousness and the Cognitive-Emotional System 1

Does the Mysterious "Wave of Death" Mark the
Critical Divide Between Life and Death? 57

.

This book is dedicated to all the teachers, professors, and mentors who inspired me to pursue my scientific interests with confidence, passion, and persistence. It is also dedicated to my Lord Jesus Christ without whose guiding light I would not be able to find the truth+

© BINDER FOUNDATION | WWW.DRMICHAELBINDER.COM

ARTICLE 1

Rethinking the Mind-Brain Duality:

Converging Lines of Evidence Shed New Light on the Anatomy of Consciousness and the Cognitive-Emotional System

Abtsract: Throughout the ages, the phenomenon of consciousness has been a subject of intense philosophical and scientific debate. Short of sufficient evidence that the mind is an entity distinct from the brain, the assumption has been that all mental and emotional processes—the essential elements of consciousness—are products of complex brain function. However, converging lines of clinical, anatomical, and biophysical evidence point back to the mind being an independent, self-governing entity as postulated by some of the world's greatest philosophers, scientists, and thinkers. Brave new insights into the anatomical and functional relationship between the mind and the brain provide logical explanations for a number of unexplained psychological, neurological, and experiential phenomena and may improve our understanding of mental and neurological illnesses. In this substantiative report, the functional anatomy of the human mind will be discussed, the point of interface between the mind and the brain will be deduced, and the means by which the mind interacts with the brain at the biophysical level will be theorized. This will be followed by a discussion of how these new insights help answer some of the toughest questions in the fields of psychology, psychiatry, and neurology.

1.0 Introduction

Since antiquity, theologians, philosophers, and scientists have pondered the inner workings of the human mind. As the brain became recognized as the organ of thought, there ensued a growing debate about whether the mind was an entity distinct from the brain or purely a product of complex brain function. Some of history's most renowned thinkers, including Socrates, Plato, Descartes, Popper, and Eccles believed that the essence of the mind was different than that of the brain. The first to write extensively about the mind–brain duality was the 16th century pioneer in mathematics, science, and metaphysics René Descartes. Descartes believed that the mind, though working closely with the brain, had a completely different nature than the brain. Like many of those before him, he contended that the substance of the mind had to be different than that of the brain because the mind was rational, whereas the brain was physical. He also believed that the mind was able to function independent of the brain and the rest of the body. However, these ideas gave rise to the historic mind-body problem: how could the mind and the brain communicate with each other if their natures were different? Short of an answer to that historic question, the mind-body duality has largely been replaced by the more accepted idea that the mind is purely a product of complex brain function.

In recent years, however, there have been a burgeoning number of reports of persons claiming to have left their physical bodies after being pronounced clinically dead[1,2]. These reports, which have now grown into the millions from around the world, have rekindled the debate about the mind-brain duality of the cognitive-emotional system. In addition, there are a number of phenomena in psychology, psychiatry, and neurology that are difficult to explain apart from a duality of mind and brain, such as memory storage and retrieval, the psychophysiological distinction between conscious and unconscious thoughts, the modulation of attention, stress-induced kindling of the brain, the psychophysiology of psychiatric disorders, psychotic states, the paradoxical effects of psychedelic drugs, the psychophysiology of psychological defense mechanisms, dissociative states, the differential response to an identical stimulus in different contexts, phantom limb and phantom sound syndromes, Savant syndrome, the split localization of thoughts and emotions, subliminal perception, time dilation, the "life review," near-death experiences (NDEs), and the critical divide between life and death.

This substantiative report will challenge the widely-held idea that the mind is merely a product of complex brain function and attempt to show that, on the contrary, the mind is the driver of brain function and the seat of cognition, attention, will, memory, and moral reasoning. Next, it will draw on major advances in neurology, biology, and physics to propose a possible solution the historic mind-body problem and attempt to elucidate the anatomical, functional, and biophysical relationship between the mind and the brain. The report will then conclude with a discussion of how the mind-brain duality of the cognitive-emotional system helps answer some of the most challenging questions in the fields of psychology, psychiatry, and neurology.

2.0 Neuropsychiatric Observations

In the 1950s, pioneering neurosurgeon Wilder Penfield found that different thoughts, different emotions, and different sensations could be triggered by stimulating different parts of the brain with an electric probe[3]. Fast-forward to the 21st century, and more profound effects on the cognitive-emotional system are being achieved without even touching the brain. Through a technique called Repetitive Transcranial Magnetic Stimulation (rTMS), doctors are learning to treat various psychiatric and neurological disorders by positioning a magnetic coil near the scalp-line, and in another technique called "optogenetics," neuroscientists are stimulating individual brain cells with the energy of light[4]. The success of these techniques demonstrates that electromagnetic energy, whether through an electric probe, a magnetic coil, or visible light, can stimulate the brain.

There is, however, a very natural way to stimulate the brain, that being through the development of cognitive-emotional stress. It is well-known that severe or chronic emotional stress can stimulate increased brainwave activity and cause electrochemical disturbances in the brain[5]. Hypothetically, symptoms such as anxiety, depression, and irritability develop when the associated circuits become pathologically hyperactive[6-10]. Though the mechanism by which stress stimulates the brain remains elusive, a large body of literature contends that stress is a subjective experience rather than a purely physiological one[11]. This leads to the hypothesis that the mind (consciousness), which is what experiences the stress, can act as an internal pulse generator that stimulates the brain. The most plausible means by which this could occur would be the same as that by which an electric probe, a magnetic coil, and visible light can stimulate the brain—electromagnetic energy (Figure 1). This hypothesis could also explain how conscious volition directs the movements of the body and how cognitive-emotional stress can have such a powerful influence on virtually every physiological function of the body.

MIND AS INTERNAL PULSE GENERATOR

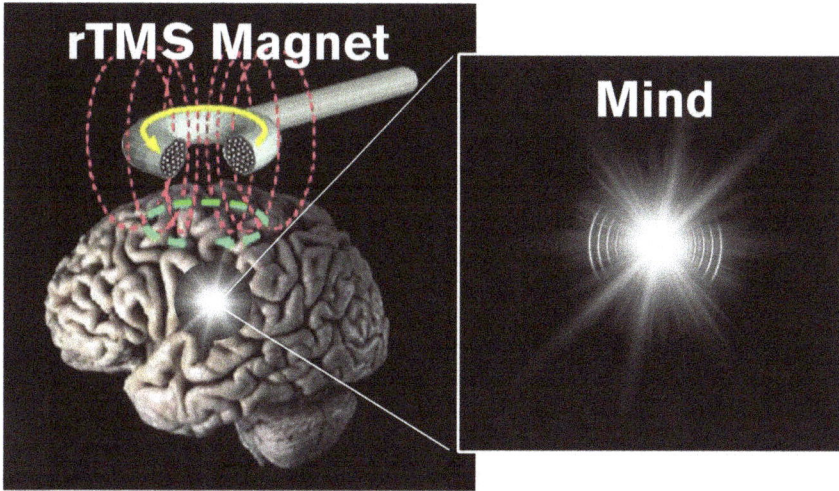

Figure 1. Like a generator magnet in rTMS, the mind (white burst), acting as an internal pulse generator, could, in theory, magnetically induce electrical activity in the brain. Likewise, electrical activity in the brain could magnetically induce activity in the mind, thus providing a mechanism by which the mind and the brain could interact with each other. © Michael R. Binder, MD.

The idea that the mind could act as an internal pulse generator leads to a number of challenging questions, such as: what is the nature of the mind? what does the mind look like? how does the mind communicate with the brain? what are the functions of the mind in relation to the brain? Where is the mind located in relation to the brain?

Fielding these questions would shed new light on the relationship between the mind and the brain and broaden our understanding of a number of unexplained psychophysiological and neuropsychiatric phenomena.

2.1   What is the Nature of the Mind?

Based on the hypothesis that the mind is an internal pulse generator, its nature would have to be energetic—spiritual. Consistent with this hypothesis, human beings possess a number of attributes that are likewise of a spiritual nature. These include thoughts, feelings, attention, will, creativity, morality, wisdom, understanding, love, and many other attributes that are not of a physical nature. We also have an innate desire to care for and protect ourselves. This too is of a spiritual nature. None of these attributes can be ascribed to the brain or other parts of the physical body any more than the parts of the physical body can be ascribed to our spiritual nature. What can be done, however, is to ascribe each attribute to the part of a human being to which its nature belongs. To the mind can be ascribed the spiritual attributes, and to the body can be ascribed the physical attributes that make us human.

Although the mind is notoriously difficult to define materially or anatomically, it can be defined by its attributes. The attributes of the mind can be divided into two functional categories: those that relate to the preservation of self (i.e., our carnal nature), and those that relate to the preservation of society (i.e., our moral nature). Our carnal nature is characterized by carnal instincts that help ensure our survival in the flesh. These include the perception of pain, temperature, touch, hunger, fatigue, and a variety of other sensations that help ensure our physical well-being. The emotions that these sensations produce, some of which are pleasant and others of which are unpleasant, are also part of our carnal nature. Our moral nature is characterized by moral instincts that help us grow spiritually and contribute to the common good. These include honesty, patience, kindness, forgiveness, and other virtues that, when practiced through the gift of will, form the basis of love. Our moral nature gives rise to peace, joy, shame, guilt, and other emotions that stem from our moral instincts just as our carnal nature gives rise to fear, anger, pleasure, excitement, and other emotions that stem from our carnal instincts. The very fact that the mind has this duality of natures is further evidence that it is more than just a manifestation of brain function, for how can one organ, being made of the same components throughout, have two different natures?

In distinction to the mind, the brain is a biological computer that gathers information from the body, integrates it, and presents it to the mind. The mind, acting as an internal pulse generator, theoretically responds by sending messages back to the brain. The dialogue between the mind and the brain is what would allow a person to process information within the context of the physical world.

2.2   What Does the Mind Look Like?

As an energy body, the mind would not be expected to be visible unless its vibrations were in the visible spectrum, and clearly they are not because no part of the mind has ever been seen. Yet the mind makes its presence known by the stimulatory effects that it has on the brain[5-7,12,13].

2.3   How Does the Mind Communicate With the Brain?

The answer to this historic question is suggested by modern advances in biology, chemistry, and physics. Like all forms of energy, the mind would be expected to induce magnetic fields, and those magnetic fields would be expected to change as a person thinks and emotes. Likewise, the neurons of the brain induce magnetic fields as charged ions flow across their respective channels during the process of depolarization, repolarization, and chemical transmission[14-16]. Hence, the mind and the brain are poised to communicate in the same language—electromagnetic energy (Figure 2). In theory, the mind could influence the brain via its magnetic fields, and the brain could influence the mind via its magnetic fields.

Had the philosophers, scientists, and thinkers of the past had the scientific information that we have today, their theories about the duality of mind and brain may have been received more favorably. However, as late as the 18th century, the understanding of electricity was still rudimentary, cellular biology was just being discovered, and the properties of electromagnetism were still unknown. Hence, the historic mind–body problem could not be solved.

MIND–BRAIN INTERACTIONS

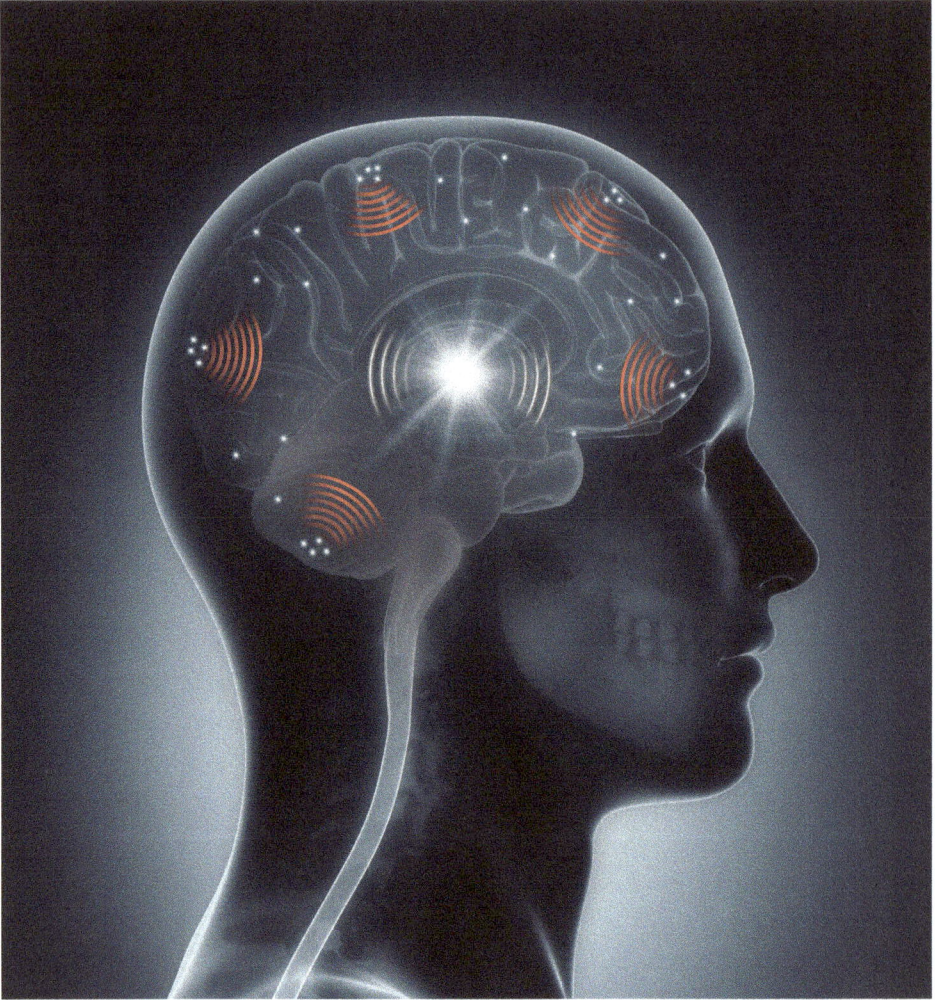

Figure 2. Schematic illustration of mentally–induced magnetic fields (white radiations) and neurologically–induced magnetic fields (red radiations). Based on the laws of electromagnetism, mentally–induced magnetic fields could stimulate the production of neurologically–induced magnetic fields and vice–versa. Yet only when the two became synchronized would the mind, owing to the slower–functioning brain, be able to experience the content in the protracted form that has traditionally been referred to as "consciousness"—"the perception of what passes in a man's own mind" (John Locke: Essay Concerning Human Understanding, 1690). © Michael R. Binder, MD.

2.4   What are the Functions of the Mind in Relation to the Brain?

From a dualistic perspective, the mind would be the head of the body, the executor that would tell the body what to say, what to do, and what to think. The brain would be the transducer that would translate these messages into electrical signals that animate and train the body. It would be through the brain's electrical system that the mind would be able to order muscles to contract and influence a wide variety of autonomic functions including heart rate, blood pressure, digestion, elimination, and endocrine function. Because the brain also relays information from the body to the mind, the brain would be the means by which the body would have an equally powerful influence on mental processes.

2.5   Where is the Mind Located?

This last question is the most challenging because the mind, being both invisible and subtle, cannot be located by physical inspection, nor can it be easily distinguished from the energy vibrations that are produced by the physical body. Locating the mind also forces us to look deeper into the essence of the mind, which again is difficult because so little is known about this aspect of it. However, a detailed analysis of the neurological system in conjunction with related clinical observations provides enough mapping information to localize the mind (or at least the primary sphere of its influence) with a fairly high degree of precision.

3.0 The Cockpit of the Mind Deep Within the Brain

In order for the brain to serve the mind effectively, it would have to funnel all sensory input to the mind on a continual basis. Furthermore, all of the information would have to be made available to the mind simultaneously on a moment-to-moment basis. For example, in order to execute a tennis shot, the mind would have to know where the ball was, where the racket was relative to the ball, where the opponent was, where the fault line was, and many other pieces of information in the form of a snapshot or fully constructed puzzle. That means that the projections of neural circuits that bore the pieces of the puzzle would have to converge somewhere in the brain.

There is a place in the brain where that occurs, and it occurs in only one place—the thalamus. The thalamus is strategically positioned to receive information from nearly every part of the body and present it to the mind simultaneously. It is also strategically positioned to project select pieces of the information to widespread areas of the brain for higher processing, and then receive the information back again for further review by the mind (Figure 3). This direct, two-way communication network between the thalamus and the higher centers of the brain is represented structurally by the vertical orientation of the columns of the neocortex

Looking more closely at the thalamus, one finds that a portion of the surface is comprised of a sheath of neurons called the *thalamic reticular nucleus (TRN)*. All neuronal projections from the thalamus to the cerebral cortex pass through it, as do all reverse projections from the cortex to the thalamus[17]. In addition, for all groups of neurons whose projections pass through a specific section of the TRN en-route to the cerebral cortex, there is a reverse projection from the cortex that passes through the same section of the TRN[17]. Thus, the cells of the TRN are topographically arranged to form a map of the body that corresponds to the same map in the cerebral cortex. This makes the TRN a spatially arranged hub that is capable of modulating nearly all of the informational traffic that is being processed by the brain (Figure 4).

Though once thought to be a passive relay center, more recent studies have found that the thalamus is heavily involved in sensory processing and, like a patrol officer directing traffic at a busy intersection, coordinates the flow of information through various parts of the brain for higher processing. For example, when light stimulates the retina of the eye, the information is relayed to the thalamus before it is sent to the visual cortex for higher processing (Figure 3). The same occurs with

ANATOMICAL AND FUNCTIONAL RELATIONSHIP BETWEEN THE MIND, THE THALAMUS, AND OTHER PARTS OF THE BRAIN

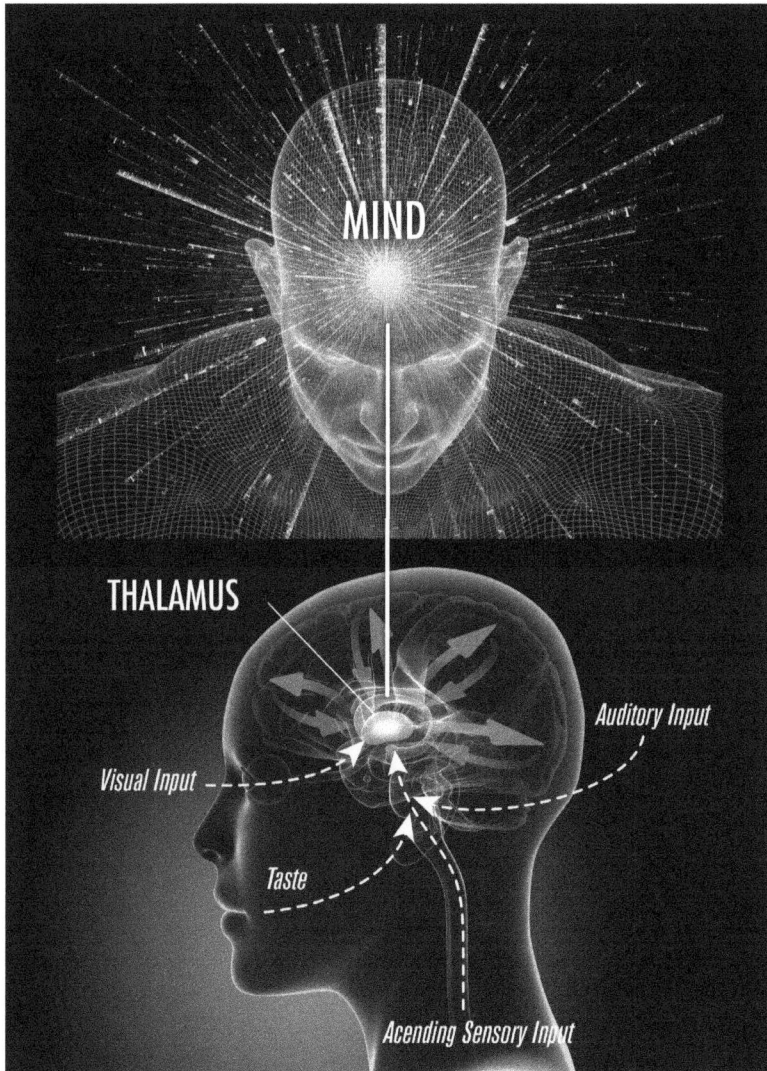

FIGURE 3. The upper image depicts mental energy (white burst) emanating from the area where the thalamus (lower image) is located. The lower image also illustrates the bidirectional flow of electrical traffic between the thalamus and various areas of the brain as the information is being processed psychophysiologically. © Michael R. Binder, MD.

INTERACTIONS BETWEEN THE MIND, THE THALAMUS, AND THE BRAIN

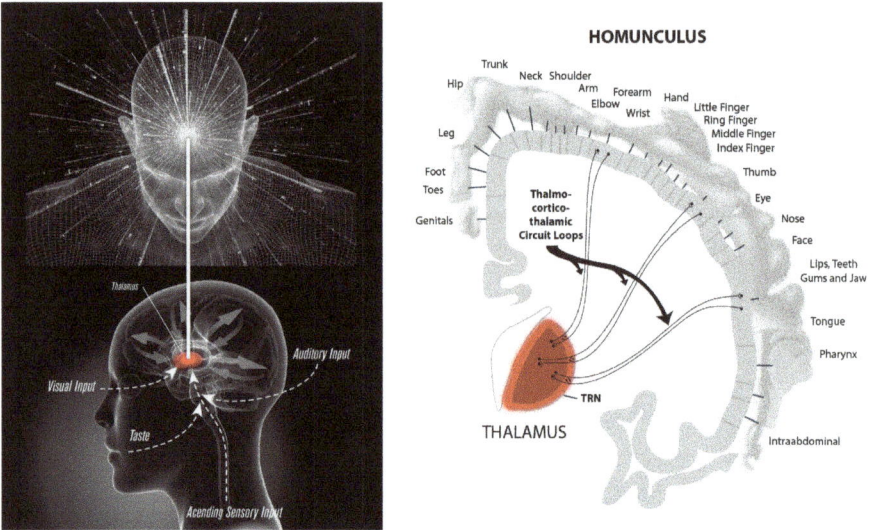

HOMUNCULUS

Figure 4: Schematic illustration of the mind seated deep within the brain. Hypothetically, the mind regulates neurological activity by directly influencing the thalamic reticular nucleus, through which all thalamocortical and corticothalamic circuit loops pass to create a thalamic homunculus that corresponds to the cortical homunculus. © *Michael R. Binder, MD.*

sound, taste, touch, and almost all other sensory inputs. But in addition to modulating the flow of information to the cortex, the thalamus continues to be a part of the conversation as the information is being processed. In a set of elegant imaging experiments, Drs. Brian Theyel and Daniel Llano found that severing the connections between two separate but communicating parts of the cortex in the mouse brain did not prevent the communication from occurring. Instead, communication continued via circuit loops between the two different parts of the cortex and the thalamus[18] (Figure 4). This shows that corticothalamocortical circuit loops are involved in the higher processing of information. Another observation demonstrates how important these circuit loops are. When one eye is continuously deprived of visual input early in development, there is a decrease in the number of cortical neurons responding to the blinded eye together with an increase in the number of cortical neurons responding to the seeing eye. Eventually, the imbalance of visual stimulation results in a reduction in the number of cortical inputs from the thalamic regions relaying information from the closed eye together with an enhancement in the number of inputs from the thalamic regions relaying information from the seeing eye. These changes are accompanied by a remodeling of the related horizontal connections in the cortex[19]. This indicates that corticothalamocortical circuit loops are not just alternative pathways; rather, they are essential to normal cortical function. Other research has found that, in addition to processing visual input, the thalamus coordinates cortical synchrony, executive function, sensory-motor activity, goal-directed behavior, levels of arousal, emotional states, behavioral flexibility, and the storage of memories[20,21]. Additionally, gamma-band oscillations in the cortex, which are known to be related to the binding of stimulus features as a whole, are concurrent with thalamic gamma activity at discrete conscious events.

Clearly, the thalamus is the operational cockpit of the brain. But can you imagine a group of cells making all our decisions for us? Muscle cells don't do that; heart cells don't; stomach cells don't. So how could one assume that brain cells, which are made of the same building blocks as these other cells, make our decisions for us? Such a thing would make us mindless automatons whose lives were dictated by the whims of neurological reflexes and spontaneous biochemical reactions. Clearly, it is the human mind that makes human decisions; but I propose that as the mind picks and chooses, the associated magnetic fields influence the cells of the TRN, which in turn influence virtually all of the electrical traffic in the brain. The continuous input of the mind is what theoretically distinguishes willful thinking from neurological reflexes.

The pioneering work of Anne Treisman and her colleagues[22-24], supported more recently by a set of elegant experiments by Julesz[25,26] and Bergen and Julesz[27] has suggested that there is an "attentional searchlight" that scans and selects information coming into the TRN[17]. According to the authors, it does this by stimulating select assemblies of cells in the TRN. The metaphorical searchlight is not proposed to light up areas of a completely dark landscape but rather, like a searchlight at dusk, is thought to illuminate those parts of a dimly lit landscape that are of particular interest to it.

The metaphorical searchlight can be none other than the human mind as it scans information coming into the TRN. Like a pilot seated in the cockpit of an airplane, the mind selects those inputs that it deems to be most important and continues to modulate them as they undergo higher processing in the corresponding areas of the brain. The shell-like structure of the reticular nucleus forms the thalamic cockpit, and the cells of the reticular nucleus constitute the cockpit's control panel. From this strategic position, the mind interacts with magnetic fields that are induced by the electrical traffic that enters and exits the thalamus. As the mind perceives the information, it can highlight select inputs by shifting attention to them (Figure 5). Those inputs that are not selected tend to be inhibited by TRN collaterals, which are known to be GABAergic[28,29]. Anatomically, the separation of the two halves of the thalamus by the aqueous third ventricle likely helps prevent left-right confusion as mentally-induced magnetic fields interact with neurologically-induced magnetic fields.

Further evidence that the thalamus is the operational cockpit of the mind is the profound effect that various manipulations of thalamic activity can have on consciousness. For example, when GABA agonists are injected into the intralaminar nucleus of the thalamus in rats, there is a slowing of the EEG, and the animals fall asleep (Alkire et al., 2008). This can rapidly be reversed by injecting a small amount of nicotine into the same part of the thalamus[30]. In theory, the nicotine provides the cholinergic input that would normally be provided by the upper brainstem and basal forebrain, areas that are known to be important in stimulating arousal[31,32]. In humans, even mild damage to the thalamus can result in a vegetative state[33]. Conversely, deep brain stimulation of the thalamus has been found to be of some benefit in rousing patients from a minimally conscious state[34,35].

Moreover, the most consistent regional effect of general anesthetics is a reduction of thalamic metabolism, and, conversely, a restoration of

PROPOSED CIRCUITRY OF THE MIND-BRAIN INTERFACE

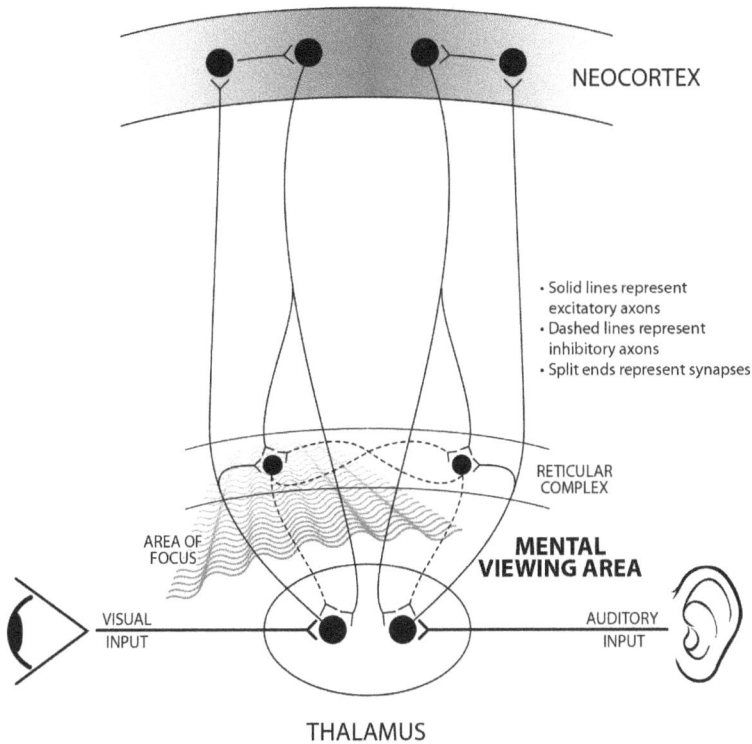

NEOCORTEX

- Solid lines represent excitatory axons
- Dashed lines represent inhibitory axons
- Split ends represent synapses

RETICULAR COMPLEX

AREA OF FOCUS

MENTAL VIEWING AREA

VISUAL INPUT

AUDITORY INPUT

THALAMUS

Figure 5. Schematic illustration of the human mind (wavy grid) scanning information coming into the TRN at the mind-brain interface. Input from the eyes, ears, integument, and other sensory organs is relayed directly to the corresponding nuclei of the thalamus (bottom center). From there the signals are sent to the corresponding areas of the cerebral cortex for higher processing before looping back to the corresponding nuclei of the thalamus. Both going and coming, collaterals from these informational tracts synapse with target cells of the reticular nucleus, thereby creating a mental touchscreen through which the mind can monitor and modulate nearly all of the information that is being processed by the brain. Note that the reticular neurons are inhibitory, thus allowing the TRN to act as a circuit-breaker that keeps the mind from becoming distracted by information that it does not intentionally select. Adapted from Crick, 1984: "Function of the thalamic reticular complex: The searchlight hypothesis." © Michael R. Binder, MD.

consciousness is typically heralded by a resumption of functional connectivity between the thalamus and the cerebral cortex[30]. In theory, the return of thalamocortical function provides the mind with the neurological input that it needs to wake up and resume its normal dialogue with the brain. This in turn allows it to regain awareness of the body and its surroundings.

Here again, a distinction must be made between corporeal consciousness, which is dependent on the body, and incorporeal consciousness, which by definition is independent of the body. What theoretically makes consciousness dependent on the body when the mind is seated in the thalamic cockpit is that it is insulated from the outside world by the brain and skull, having no access to sensory input save that which is conveyed by neurological signals. In the absence of these signals, it simply falls asleep. This idea is supported by the observation that the natural process of falling asleep is typically initiated by a decrease in sensory input and inhibitory mechanisms that divert neurological signals away from the mind–brain interface[36-38]. In theory, the same loss of signaling could be brought about by neurological abnormalities that prevented or interfered with the production of the magnetic fields that would normally stimulate wakefulness. If the disruption were brief, as in the case of a mild brain injury, the loss of consciousness would be temporary. If it were prolonged, as in the case of a severe brain injury, the mind would remain in a pathological state of sleep that could be described as "coma." The idea that the mind is simply asleep when there is a severe and persistent disruption of communication between the mind and the brain is supported by the observation that deep sleep and coma are virtually identical both clinically and electrophysiologically[39].

Now then, if the mind were to separate from the brain, as it theoretically does during the transition from life to death, it would have continuous access to the outside world and would presumably remain awake continuously. This idea is corroborated by the growing number of near–death testimonials in which experiencers say that during their NDE they were fully conscious and alert, apparently without any fatigue or need for sleep despite documented evidence that they were deeply unconscious while they were said to be outside their physical body. Then again, even when the mind receives too much stimulation while in the thalamic cockpit, it tends to remain awake continuously, thus explaining why nearly all psychiatric disorders, which are hypothesized to be rooted in neuronal hyperexcitability[6-8,40], include the symptom of insomnia.

The idea that the mind, as an entity distinct from the brain, can "fall asleep" also explains the peculiar separation between wakefulness and awareness that is characteristic of absence seizures. During an absence episode, the affected individual remains awake, yet loses consciousness. This phenomenon would be difficult to explain if consciousness were merely a synthesis of neurologically-induced magnetic fields because such a conceptualization would not allow for wakefulness to occur without any awareness of being awake. If, on the other hand, the mind were an entity distinct from the brain, it could in theory be kept awake by the seizure activity, yet without any comprehension of it due to the loss of intelligibility that would occur when normal signaling became hypersynchronized. In a clever study by Casali et al.[41], conscious perception was induced by stimulating specific brain areas with transcranially-generated magnetic fields. In accordance with Faraday's law, the magnetic fields caused current to flow in various circuits of the brain just as it does when a person thinks and emotes. However, conscious perception, as reported by the test subjects, was associated with distributed, non-uniform magnetic fields as opposed to those that were either localized and non-integrated, or widespread and uniform, as might be expected during epileptic seizures or slow wave sleep. This suggests that it is the intelligibility of the magnetic fields rather than their source that determines their ability to be perceived as meaningful. The theoretical reason that intelligible signals generally involve widespread areas of the brain is that the brain signaling must be just as intelligible as the signals that the mind sends to it, and such detailed signaling would logically involve contributions from various different neurons and circuits. Based on the ability of intelligible magnetic fields to illicit intelligible responses from the conscious mind, Dr. Casali and his team are studying ways to use the evoked activity as a means of determining whether a minimally responsive patient is actually conscious.

The idea that the mind has the capacity to think and emote independent of the brain and body is further supported by the findings of Nakajima and Halassa[42], who concluded that although the thalamus regulates functional connectivity within and between cortical regions, it does not necessarily determine the content of a cognitive process. Nor can consciousness be localized to the cerebral cortex, as children who are born without a cortex are conscious[43], and in their pioneering work, Penfield and others found that awareness of self and environment were fully preserved as they surgically removed relatively large areas of the cortex to treat refractory seizures[31,43]. The difficulty pinpointing which brain structure, area, or function mediates corporeal consciousness suggests that neurological activity, though necessary to support corporeal consciousness, is an epiphenomenon and that there must be an independent observer who perceives the information that is conveyed by neurological activity, considers it, and then drives neurological activity as it processes the information. I propose that that observer is the human mind.

4.0 Mental Modulation of Thalamic Output

Although TRN collaterals are largely (if not entirely) inhibitory, specialized burst activity allows them to enhance the activation of select neural networks when stimulated. The mechanism by which this occurs is based on the unique physiology of thalamic neurons. Elegant studies on thalamic slices from the guinea pig[44-46] have confirmed that when hyperpolarized thalamic neurons are stimulated, they respond by producing a single spike (or short burst of rapid spikes) followed by a brief period during which they are unresponsive to continued stimulation. Thus, when the mind turns its attention to a point of interest, the excitatory phase of neuronal activation initiates a wave of inhibition that turns down irrelevant information, while the refractory phase allows activity in select circuits to be turned up (Figure 5). In this way, the TRN allows the mind to scan the information coming into the thalamus, highlight select inputs, and then shift attention to other areas of potential interest. This modulatory mechanism has been proposed by several investigators including Anne Treisman, who was awarded the National

Medal of Science in 2013, and Francis Crick, who co-discovered the molecular structure of DNA.

The idea that the thalamus functions as a cockpit through which the mind can monitor and control the body is supported by the following five observations:

1. The thalamus has reciprocal connections to all areas of the cerebral cortex. This, taken together with the fact that the thalamus is the hub of sensory input, places it in the position necessary to act as a vehicle through which the mind can monitor the entire body, decide what to think about, and control the body by directing neurological activity according to the dictates of the will.

2. A specific thalamic nucleus (the TRN) is able to regulate virtually all cerebral activity via inhibitory collaterals, and these collaterals are theoretically under the influence of the mind.

3. The degree of modulation of thalamic activity is positively correlated with the subjective feeling of mental effort invested in maintaining concentration[47].

4. Emotional processing stimulates the brain more strongly than cognitive processing[48]. The rapid fall-off in magnetic field strength that is described by Coulomb's law makes this distinction relevant in locating the point of interface between the mind and the brain and is consistent with the idea that the thalamus, which is in the heart of the limbic system, is the cockpit of the mind (Figure 6).

5. Disruption of signaling to, from, or within the thalamus results in a loss of corporeal consciousness[30,33,49,50].

Taken together, these observations provide compelling evidence that the thalamus is the focal point of interaction between the mind and the brain; it is the seat of corporeal consciousness that Descartes was looking for.

SPACIAL RELATIONSHIP BETWEEN THE PROPOSED LOCATION OF THE MIND AND VARIOUS BRAIN STRUCTURES

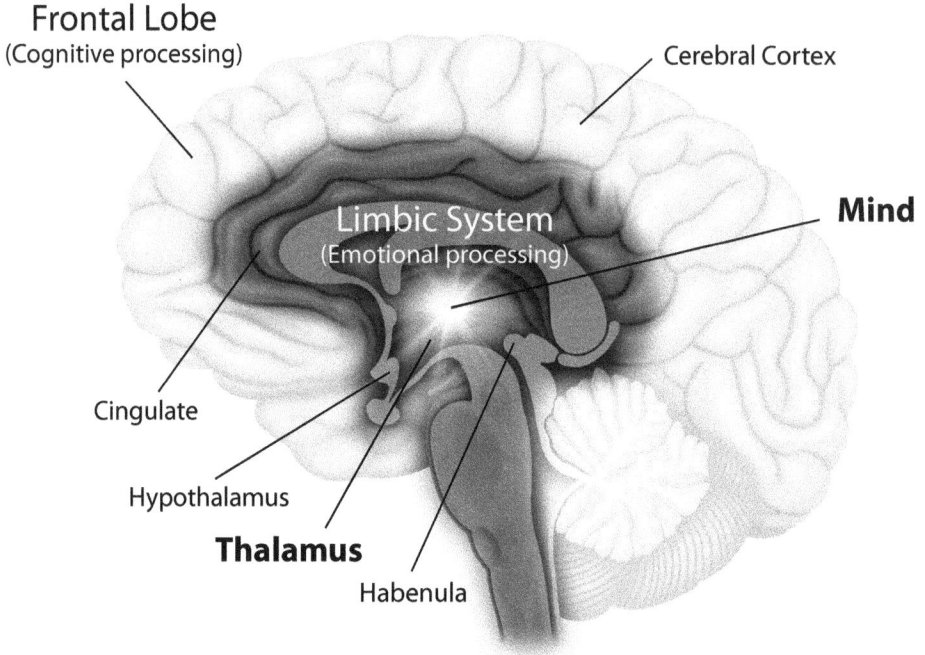

Figure 6. Relative proximities of the limbic system (darkly shaded area) and the cognitive and other systems of the brain (lightly shaded area) to the thalamus, the proposed cockpit of the mind. © Michael R. Binder, MD.

5.0 Practical Application of the Mind–Brain Duality of the Cognitive–Emotional System

Having answered the five basic questions about the mind in relation to the brain, let us turn our attention to how a duality of mind and brain can help answer some of the most challenging questions in the fields of psychology, psychiatry, and neurology.

5.1   Psychophysiology of Memory Storage and Retrieval

From the perspective of the mind-brain duality of the cognitive-emotional system, selective attention, thoughts, emotions, choices, and the memory of them are obligate functions of the mind. However, just as a computer and internet service are needed to interact with the cyber world, a brain and body are needed for the mind to interact with the physical world. In theory, the mind interacts with the brain and body through an anatomical and functional alignment that is an extension of the alignment between the brain and body. For example, if one were observing something, light would activate receptors in the eye that were specifically designed to respond to visual input. From there, sensory nerve fibers would relay the neural code to the mind-brain interface, where the associated magnetic fields would influence the mind with the same specificity as the electromagnetic rays that stimulated them. Conversely, if one were thinking about something, the magnetic fields generated by the mind would induce electrical activity in vibration-specific neurons and circuits at the mind-brain interface[51,52] and the associated areas of the brain[53-55]. The coupling between specific vibrational frequencies of the mind and specific neurons and circuits of the brain would occur in a way analogous to the coupling between specific types of sensory input to the body and specific sensory receptors and pathways, such as those for light, sound, and touch[56]. Thus far, some 721 different types of neurons have been reconstructed from 317 brain regions, and the number of circuits in the brain is virtually incomprehensible *(http://neuromorpho.org/. Accessed 5/16/18).*

As previous stated, when specialized neurons were stimulated by specific mental processes, they would fire in burst patterns that corresponded to the associated vibrational frequencies. Because these bursts of activity and their spike trains would propagate for a longer period of time than mental impulses, which, being electromagnetic, would be lightning-fast, the magnetic fields that they induced would have the effect of sustaining thoughts and emotions. They would also have the effect of increasing the strength of the magnetic fields, thus increasing the ease with which they could be perceived and held in consciousness by the mind.

Therein lies the distinction between conscious and unconscious thoughts: unconscious thoughts become conscious when they successfully activate the corresponding neural network[57]. Once a thought becomes conscious, the mind can edit that thought by deciding to think about it in a new way. As a part of that process, the brain would undergo subtle physiological and structural changes in accordance with the new way that the mind had decided to use that thought and the new associations it made to it. The more the mind thought about something in the new way, the more the brain would reconfigure itself to the new way of thinking and the more likely it would be to regenerate the corresponding neural code in response to a related mental impulse. In other words, the more likely it would be to be "remembered" (Figure 7). What in theory would create the sense of a thought "popping" into consciousness would be the sudden synchronization of a neurologically-derived magnetic field with a mentally-derived magnetic field. Because the brain is able to process information at a top speed of approximately 100 meters/sec, which is about 3,000,000 times slower than the lightning-fast mind would be able to process information, most mental processing would not be expected to reach conscious awareness (Figure 7). Consciousness in this context could more aptly be referred to as "corporeal consciousness" because it would occur in synchrony with the brain. This would be in contrast to "incorporeal consciousness," which would occur independent of the brain and body.

Since energy is indestructible, the mind presumably never forgets anything that it perceives. In contrast, the subtle changes that occur in the brain each time that a specific circuit (or set of circuits) is activated are subject to further modification and decay. Hence, these changes must be reinforced if they are to be regenerated in response to a related mental impulse. When we

CONSCIOUS AND UNCONSCIOUS THOUGHTS

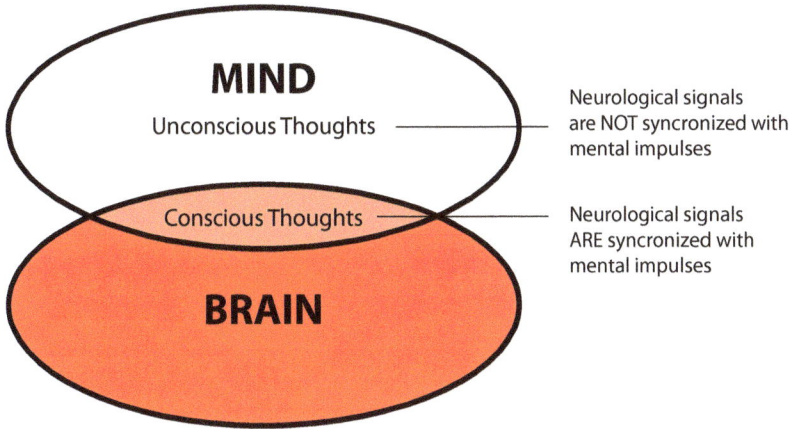

MIND
Unconscious Thoughts —————————— Neurological signals are NOT syncronized with mental impulses

Conscious Thoughts —————————— Neurological signals ARE syncronized with mental impulses

BRAIN

Figure 7. Because the brain is a much slower processor than the mind, very little mental processing would be expected to occur consciously. © *Michael R. Binder, MD.*

find ourselves struggling to remember something that we know that we know, what is apparently happening is that we (our mind) is trying to draw our brain into synch with the vibrational pattern that corresponds to the memory that we are trying to consciously recollect. Neural oscillations originating in the thalamus sweep through the brain forty times per second, theoretically drawing different neural circuits into synch with mental intensions[58,59].

In theory then, memories are stored in the mind, though the conscious recollection of them requires a synchronization between mentally-induced magnetic fields and neurologically-induced magnetic fields. As alluded to earlier, thoughts, feelings, and memories could also be precipitated by spontaneous neural signaling, which would explain why a long-forgotten name, feeling, or event can suddenly become conscious without any mental effort to retrieve it. It would also explain why various emotions, such as anxiety, depression, and euphoria could be experienced spontaneously if the brain became pathologically hyperactive[6,7].

5.2 Modulation of Attention

Both selective attention and attentional disorders can best be explained through a duality of mind and brain. What we call "concentration" theoretically involves a dynamic interplay between the mind and the brain in which the mind, through focused effort, stimulates activity in select populations of neurons. In the process, the mind also stimulates TRN collaterals, which, being largely inhibitory, turn down the activity of circuits that convey less relevant or competing information[17] (Figure 4). Thalamic modulation would be enhanced if one were highly interested in something because input from dopaminergic neurons, which are normally activated when one is heavily invested in what one is doing, disinhibits the reticular neurons, thereby enhancing their modulatory capacity[60]. This would explain why it normally takes less mental effort to maintain focus on things that one enjoys doing. Even if one were not enjoying a specific activity, attention could be improved through mental effort, as it would directly enhance the modulatory function of the reticular neurons (Figure 5). In extreme cases, such as when there were a perceived threat, the intensity with which the mind would stimulate the reticular neurons would be extremely high, thus optimizing focus. Another factor that would help optimize focus during fight-or-flight would be that the TRN, in addition to accepting input from dopaminergic neurons, is densely innervated by adrenergic projections from the locus coeruleus. Thus, were the sympathetic nervous system to be activated, concentration would increase dramatically. In some cases, it could even overshoot due to the combined effects of directed mental effort and adrenergic activation. This is the proposed mechanism by which crisis situations tend to cause "tunnel vision."

Then again, if excitation in the brain were spontaneously elevated, as it is hypothesized to be in psychiatric disorders[6], the relatively modest output of the reticular neurons would tend to be outweighed by the overabundance of electrical traffic through the thalamus. This would tend to impair concentration as the mind became distracted by the reverberation of various circuit loops and the thoughts and feelings to which they were linked (Figure 8). The lack of sufficient circuit–breaker activity via the TRN would cause the mind to repeatedly shift attention rather than remain focused on any one thing. This would be experienced as inattention. Furthermore, because the shifts in attention would occur so rapidly, the brain would not have enough time to fully process any one thought before the mind shifted attention to another thought. This would be experienced as distractibility. If the mind were to then decide to take action before the brain had enough time to synchronize with the relevant background information, it would be experienced as impulsivity. The means by which psychostimulants improve concentration is by enhancing the activity of dopamine and norepinephrine, both of which enhance the output of TRN collaterals. Note, however, that when taken in excess, these

PSYCHOPHYSIOLOGY OF INATTENTION

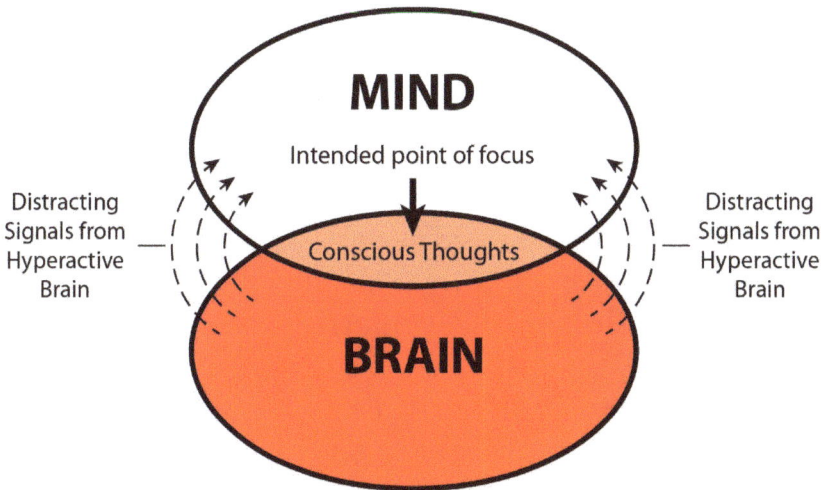

Figure 8. Dashed lines represents inappropriate messaging from the hyperactive brain, which distracts the mind from the intended point of focus.
© *Michael R. Binder, MD.*

drugs can create a physiological state akin to fight-or-flight, thus explaining the common side effect of "hyperfocus."

5.3 Stress-Induced Kindling of the Brain

Based on the proposed anatomical location of the mind deep within the core of the brain, one would expect the limbic system to be the brain area most vulnerable to stress-induced kindling both because emotional stress produces the highest levels of tension in the mind and because Coulomb's Law states that the intensity of a magnetic field is inversely proportional to the distance from its source. Indeed, the associated cells of the limbic system, which are located closest to the thalamic cockpit, would be the most strongly influenced by mental tension[16,48]. When Dr. Goddard was stimulating the amygdala of rats to determine its effects on learning, he was likely causing the animals to become emotionally distressed, an effect that would have accelerated the kindling that he was inducing electrically. This idea is supported by his observation that the number of stimulus sessions needed to induce seizures could be reduced by increasing the time interval between sessions[61]. The increased time between sessions would have allowed anticipatory anxiety to partially replace the need for electrically-induced kindling, particularly in the amygdala, which is known to be involved in the fight-or-flight response[62]. Further evidence that the mind induces kindling in the brain comes from the well-known fact that emotional stress is the most ubiquitous precipitant of psychiatric symptoms.

5.4 Psychophysiology of Psychiatric Disorders

From the perspective of the mind-brain duality, cognitive and emotion-specific magnetic fields generated by the mind induce cognitive and emotion-specific neurons in the brain to fire and send messages to other parts of the brain that are involved in the processing of those specific thoughts and feelings. Such emotion-specific neurons have now been identified using advanced in-vivo cell-monitoring and stimulus-control techniques[54]. The primary neural networking would be mediated by electrical connections between neurons, which can allow large numbers of them to fire simultaneously in response to relatively subtle mental vibrations. Associative processing would be mediated by chemical connections between neurons, which can allow information from different areas of the brain to be integrated in conjunction with ongoing input from the mind. From an electrophysiological standpoint, each time that a thought or feeling successfully activated the corresponding neural network, there would be a large increase in the strength and duration of the associated magnetic field. Again, this synchronization process is in theory what allows an unconscious thought to become conscious[57].

What theoretically distinguishes pathological neural signaling from normal signaling is that it is abnormally persistent and relatively unresponsive to mental efforts to reduce or shift attention away from it. Advanced imaging studies have found that the related brain circuits won't shut off[63,64]. Psychophysiologically, the hyperactive circuit loops would keep the mind engaged in the associated thoughts and feelings, thus creating a vicious cycle of mutual overstimulation between the mind and the brain. The resulting stress would further fuel this process, as the tension in the mind would continue to activate the specific circuit loops that were creating the stress. As previously stated, emotions stimulate the brain more strongly than cognitions, and emotional stress usually involves feelings of guilt, fear, or entrapment. This would explain why anxiety and depression, which usually accompany such feelings, are the two most common psychiatric symptoms. Then again, the circuit-specific hyperactivity could in some cases involve circuits for pleasure and excitement, thus leading to manic states. Yet in theory, the symptoms themselves are in most cases rooted in a hyperexcitability of the neurological system[6-9]. This hyperexcitability would predispose the locus of hyperactivity to migrate from one inappropriate circuit loop to another via cross-circuit activation as hyperactive feeder circuits fueled activity in inappropriate circuit loops, which, themselves

MANIC–DEPRESSIVE SWITCHING

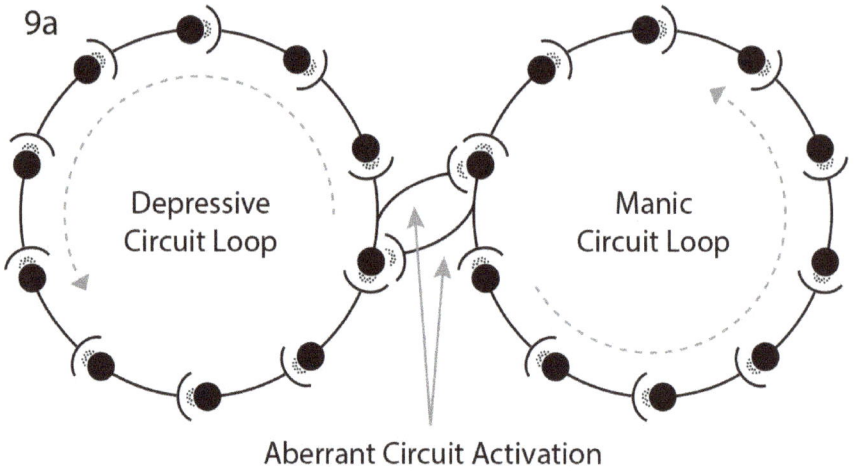

Aberrant Circuit Activation

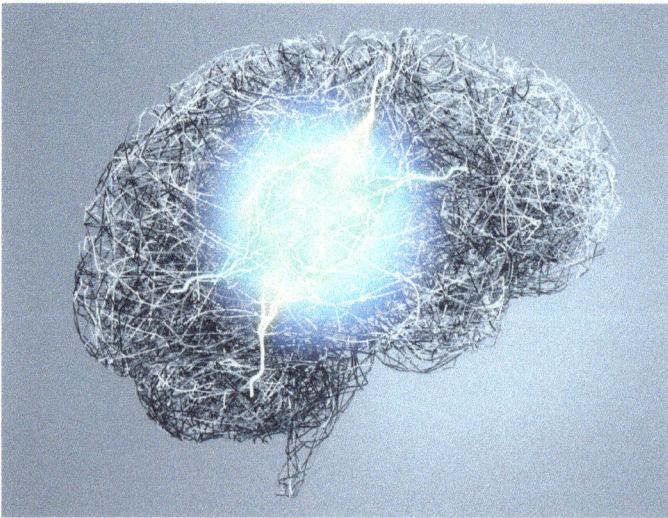

Electrical Short-Circuit

Figure 9a. Schematic illustration of one of the means by which one hyperactive circuit can aberrantly fuel hyperactivity in another circuit to cause manic-depressive switching. In the example above, the depressive circuit loop and the manic circuit loop inappropriately excite each other. This is more apt to occur in persons with neuronal hyperexcitability both because the neurological system tends to be more hyperactive and because collateral circuits, which themselves are hyperexcitable, are more easily brought to threshold by feeder circuits. Adapted from: The Multi-Circuit Neuronal Hyperexcitability Hypothesis of Psychiatric Disorders. Michael R. Binder, M.D. American Journal of Clinical and Experimental Medicine. Vol. 7, No. 1, 2019, p. 15.

Figure 9b. Schematic illustration of an electrical short-circuit occurring in the brain. © *Michael R. Binder, MD.*

being hyperexcitable, were subject to this aberrant circuit activation (Figure 9a). This process, which would be akin to a short-circuit in a wired electrical system (Figure 9b), would explain the phenomenon of bipolarity, an instability in the cognitive-emotional system that to some degree characterizes most psychiatric disorders[6,7]. The theoretical reason that insomnia is such a common symptom in psychiatric disorders is that the persistence of the heated dialogue between the mind and the brain does not allow either one of them to cool off. Presumably, psychiatric breakdowns occur when the overabundance of neural signaling becomes mentally and emotionally intolerable[6]. This conceptualization would also help explain the wide-ranging benefits of various forms of psychotherapy. By reducing mental tension, psychotherapy would help break the vicious cycle of mutual overstimulation between the mind and the brain. The neuronal hyperexcitability hypothesis of psychiatric disorders is supported by the growing body of genetic evidence that links psychiatric disorders to gene polymorphisms whose protein products fail to regulate the firing of neurons[6,65-77]. *ANK3 ankyrin 3 [Homo sapiens (human)] - Gene-NCBI Gene ID: 288. https://www.ncbi.nlm.nih.gov/gene/288. Accessed 11/1/18).*

5.5 Psychotic States

From the perspective of the mind-brain duality of the cognitive-emotional system, psychotic symptoms develop when the level of electrical activity in the sensory processing system becomes as high or higher than the level of activity that would normally be driven by input from the body's sensory organs (Figure 10). For example, overfiring of neurons in the auditory processing system would lead to the misperception that the auditory nerve were being stimulated. This would cause the person to think that the associated sounds were coming from the environment. Overfiring of neurons in the visual processing system would lead to the

PROPOSED MECHANISM OF PSYCHOTIC SYMPTOMS

(Auditory Halucinations)

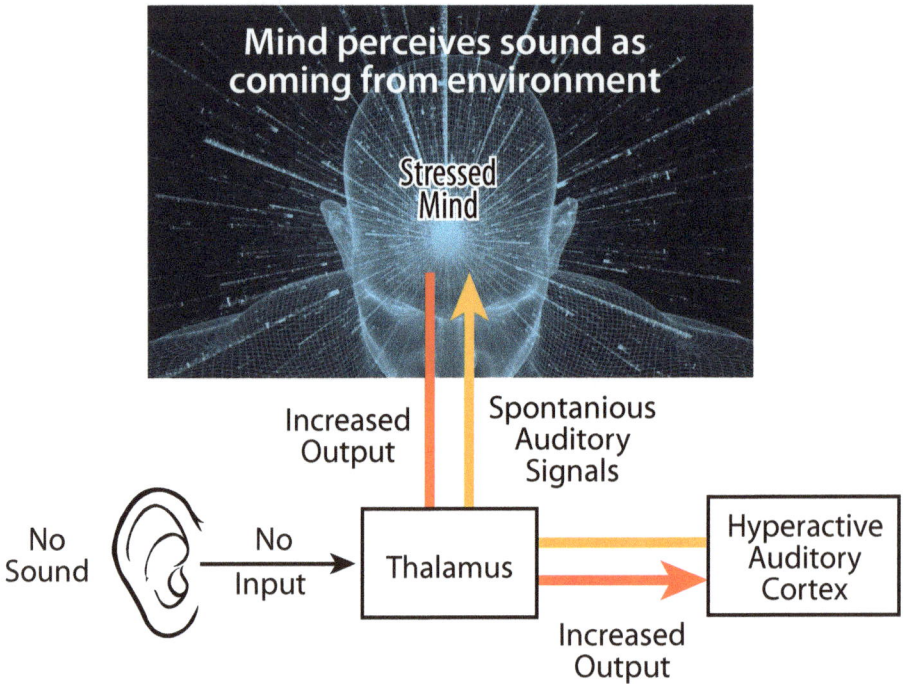

Figure 10. Diagrammatic illustration of the mechanism that is proposed to underlie auditory hallucinations and, in principle, other psychotic symptomatology. Despite a lack of auditory input, pathological hyperactivity in auditory circuits to the thalamus (the cockpit of the mind) induce local magnetic fields that cause the mind to mistakenly perceive sound as coming from the environment. Because intrapsychic stress activates brain circuits, auditory hallucinations are more likely to occur during times of stress, particularly if the brain is inherently hyperexcitable. © *Michael R. Binder, MD.*

misperception that the optic nerve were being stimulated. This would cause the person to think that the associated images were coming from the environment, etc... Although such aberrant signaling could potentially occur in anyone, it would be more likely to occur in persons with hyperexcitable neurons, such as those with schizophrenia, bipolar disorder, or some other serious mental illness[6,7]. This conceptualization is supported by a recent study that found that auditory hallucinations in schizophrenia were exaggerated versions of perceptual distortions that are not uncommonly experienced by persons who do not have schizophrenia[78]. The researchers found that the perceptual distortions were more pronounced in those test subjects whose neurons were releasing more dopamine, a neurotransmitter that is known to be involved in the processing of auditory signals[79]. Similarly, other forms of psychosis, such as paranoia and delusional thinking, would occur when internally-generated neurological signals became so intense and persistent that they were thought to reflect external events[6,40,80].

5.6 Paradoxical Effects of Psychedelic Drugs

Many users of psychedelic drugs such as LSD, DMT, and psilocybin find that their senses become expanded and their perceptions more vivid while under the influence, though real-time imaging shows a decrease in cerebral blood flow together with a reduction in neurological activity in key connector regions, such as the thalamus, the cingulate gyrus, and the prefrontal cortex[81]. There is no logical way, based on brain function alone, to explain the paradox of rising mental acuity in the face of falling neurological activity. However, from the perspective of the mind-brain duality of the cognitive-emotional system, the partial reduction in neurological activity could allow the mind to partially disengage from the brain. Were the mind to come more fully into its own, it would have a glimpse of its true capabilities, which, being of a purely spiritual nature, would be expected to be incomparably greater than those of the material-bound brain. Meanwhile the brain, being toxically prevented from processing input from the mind, would become increasingly quiescent and less metabolically active. A similar phenomenon may occur in some dream states, which would explain why dreams can sometimes be more vivid, more meaningful, and more transcendent than waking states. As the derivation of the word "psychedelic" implies (psyche, meaning "mind," and delos, meaning "manifest"), the experience of floating, the disengagement from material reality, and the dissolution of the self that may occur under the influence of psychedelic drugs suggest that the mind, under such circumstances, is at least partially disengaging from the brain and realizing its true capabilities[82-84].

5.7 Psychophysiology of Psychological Defense Mechanisms

Psychological defense mechanisms are mental efforts to avoid specific thoughts and feelings in an effort to minimize, repress, or alter one's thoughts about things that cause intolerable emotional pain. The presumed psychophysiological mechanism by which this occurs is that the mind either thinks about the emotionally painful content from a perspective that reduces intrapsychic conflict or ignores it enough to prevent the neural circuitry from synchronizing with the related mental impulses, thus preventing the content from becoming conscious.

5.8 Dissociative States

From the perspective of the mind-brain duality, dissociative states are partial or complete separations of the mind from the brain, most commonly to avoid painful thoughts, emotions, and experiences. The temporary separation would prevent neurologically induced magnetic fields from synchronizing with mentally-induced magnetic fields and vice-versa, thereby preventing the content from arising in corporeal consciousness. Though these psychic shifts may occur spontaneously at first, the experience of them can lead to a pattern of dissociating as a coping mechanism.

5.9 Differential Response to an Identical Stimulus in Different Contexts

An unexpected knock at the door in the middle of the night would naturally cause greater alarm than the same knock in the middle of the day. It would cause a greater increase in heart rate, respiratory rate, and general alertness. Yet regardless of the time, the same sound at the door would stimulate the same sensory input to the brain. Hence, the time-related difference in one's physical, emotional, and psychological response, which in most cases would be dramatic, could not possibly be explained on the basis of brain function alone. The more plausible explanation is that the same sound, though effecting a virtually identical bottom-up neurological response at either time of day, would trigger a different mental response in different contexts, thus resulting in a different top-down neurological response.

5.10 Phantom Limb and Phantom Sound Syndromes

Nearly all persons who have lost a limb due to illness or injury report painful sensations, such as burning, aching, or crushing in the place where the limb had been[85]. This is often referred to as "phantom limb pain." A similar phenomenon occurs with the auditory system in association with complete hearing loss. This condition, which involves persistent and distressing sound sensations, is known as "hyperacusis." These phenomena would be inexplicable if neurological activity alone were the generator of consciousness because the loss of a limb or the ability to hear would be expected to result in *less* rather than *more* neurological activity in the sensory centers that would normally be activated by input from the respective sensory organs. Of course, the phantom sensations could be driven by spontaneous discharges from damaged peripheral nerves[86]. However, Mercier and Sirigu found that when patients who had lost an upper limb were asked to follow with an imaginary limb the movements of a limb that had been presented to them visually, they experienced a significant reduction in phantom limb pain[87]. As illustrated in Figure 4, sensory input normally stimulates inhibitory output by TRN collaterals at the mind–brain interface. This neural inhibition would be lost were the limb to be removed, thus providing a possible explanation for phantom limb pain. Note, however, that the inhibitory output could be restored if the mind were to stimulate the same TRN collaterals (Figure 4). This is theoretically what happens when patients are asked to move as though their amputated limb were still there. The same explanation could be applied to the phenomenon of hyperacusis, wherein complete hearing loss would result in a loss of the inhibitory output that would normally be stimulated by ambient noise and other sounds from the environment. This conceptualization is supported by the observation that hyperacusis is not limited to persons with complete hearing loss. Most normal persons, when placed in a soundproof room, experience phantom sound sensations[85].

5.11 Savant Syndrome

Savants demonstrate select mental abilities that far exceed normal intellectual functioning, such as the ability to perform mathematical computations that would normally require a computer, and the ability to recite musical pieces with little or no practice. Yet, the majority of these persons have some form of mental disability or neurodevelopmental delay. This cannot be explained solely on the basis of brain function because the best that could be expected in such cases would be a preservation of some cognitive functions despite the loss of others. What apparently happens in Savant syndrome is that the individual's time, energy, and interest are funneled into fewer cognitive functions, thus providing greater mental input to those particular functions. This would naturally lead to an overdevelopment of some functions in place of others that were either lost or could not be developed due to neurological deficits in those functions. A similar phenomenon occurs in physically disabled persons who go on to develop extraordinary physical abilities using the body parts that are still functioning normally. The strong association of Savant syndrome with autism spectrum disorders, which are known to be associated with an overabundance of neurons and neuronal connections[88,89], suggests that these anomalies in brain structure may contribute to the unusual intellectual abilities of Savants[90].

5.12 Split Localization of Thoughts and Emotions

One of the most obvious forms of evidence that thoughts and emotions are not inherent functions of the brain is the self-evident fact that emotions are experienced in the chest rather than in the head, where the emotional wiring is located. All of our cognitive wiring is in the brain and, as expected, we experience our thoughts in our head. But how can one explain the fact that we experience our emotions in our chest (Figure 11)?

Not surprisingly, it was once believed that emotions emanated from the heart. However, that idea began to change with the discovery that the heart was just a pump in the chest. Of course, the brain is connected to the heart, and so one could surmise that at least some of the neural correlates of emotions could be relayed to the heart, where they are then experienced. However, the connections between the brain and the heart are severed during heart transplant surgery, and there is no evidence that those who undergo such operations experience any change in the anatomical area where they experience their emotions

From the perspective of the mind–brain duality of the cognitive-emotional system, emotions are experienced by the spiritual body, not the physical body. The observation that emotions are experienced in the chest, though the emotional wiring is in the brain, provides empirical evidence that an incorporeal entity experiences the emotions and somehow relays the related energy vibrations to the brain. What's more, the observation that the hub of those emotions is in the same area as the physical heart

RELATIONSHIP BETWEEN SPIRITUAL BODY AND PHYSICAL BODY

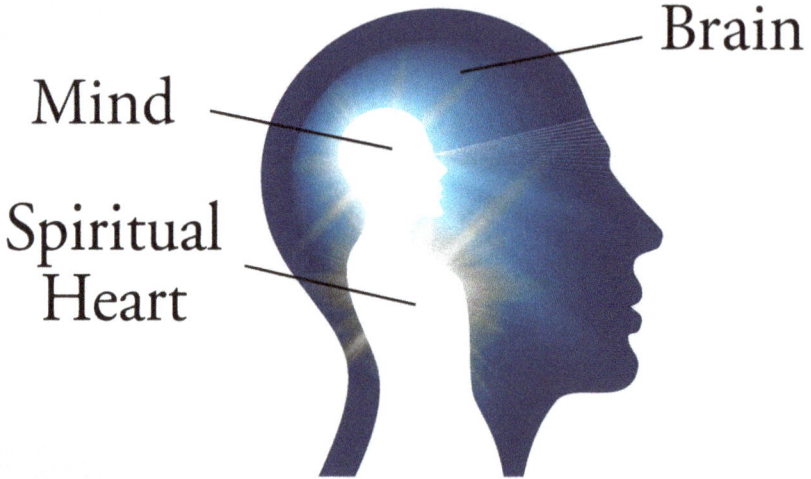

Figure 11. Schematic illustration of the spiritual body dwelling inside the physical body. As the head of the spiritual body, the mind corresponds to the brain both anatomically and functionally; likewise, the spiritual heart corresponds to the physical heart both anatomically and functionally (though not correctly positioned here). Also, just as the physical heart circulates blood to the physical body, the spiritual heart hypothetically circulates spiritual energy to the spiritual body. © *Michael R. Binder, MD.*

suggests that they may indeed be experienced in the heart—not the physical heart—but the spiritual heart. This idea, taken together with the observation that thoughts are experienced in the head, where the brain is located, suggests that the energetic essence of a human being has an anatomy that mirrors that of the physical body. If that were true, the vibrations of the spiritual heart would have to be relayed to a corresponding processing center in the head (presumably the mind) so that they could be shared with the physical brain and vice-versa, thus allowing thoughts and emotions to be integrated and processed in conjunction with bodily processes. This bidirectional flow of vibrational energy within the incorporeal or "spiritual" body could theoretically occur in a way analogous to the bidirectional flow of electrical impulses and blood within the physical body. Though difficult to prove scientifically, empirical evidence suggests that the essence of a human being is spiritual and that the physical body is merely a biological vessel that the spiritual body uses to interact with the physical world. Be that as it may, the split localization of thoughts and feelings provides further evidence that the cognitive–emotional system is an entity distinct from the brain.

5.13 Subliminal Perception

In subliminal perception, information is routed through the brain but not recognized consciously. A review of fMRI studies shows that subliminal stimuli activate specific brain regions without the individual being aware of it[91]. If the mind were merely a manifestation of brain function, this would be difficult to explain. Studies also show that subliminal stimuli can unconsciously influence subsequent thoughts, feelings, and behaviors, a finding that would be even more difficult to explain on a purely neurological basis both because the information is not committed to memory and because the individual is not consciously aware that it is having an influence.

What actually appears to be happening in subliminal perception is that both the mind and the brain are encoding the information without sufficient synchronization between the two of them to make the process conscious. Yet because both the mind and the brain encode the information, it could understandably affect subsequent thoughts, feelings, and behaviors. Moreover, because the mind presumably never forgets anything that it encodes, the effect would be expected to persist, though to a lesser extent, even after the brain had lost the electronic trace.

5.14 Time Dilation

A peculiar phenomenon that sometimes accompanies intensely emotional experiences is the perception that time and motion are slowed down. The proposed psychophysiological mechanism underlying this phenomenon, known as "time dilation," is that intensely emotional or highly captivating experiences tend to draw attention onto a single point of focus, thus causing the mind to persistently stimulate a select patch of the TRN (Figure 5). Because TRN collaterals are primarily inhibitory, peripheral input would be strongly subdued, thus further locking the mind onto a select patch of the TRN. This would tend to prevent the mind from continuing to scan the TRN as it normally would. As a result, the mind, like eyes fixed on the hands of a clock, would perceive time and events as progressing more slowly than normal.

5.15 Life Review

What presumably allows some persons to see "their whole lives flash by in front of them" is that certain extreme situations, particularly when there is a belief that death is imminent, drive a loosening of the connection between the mind and the brain, and this partial disengagement allows the mind to come more fully into its own. When allowed to function independent of the brain, the mind does not have to wait for the slower processing brain to synchronize with it. Working then at the speed of light, which is the processing speed of electromagnetic energy, it would indeed be possible for the mind to reflect on most or all of its most meaningful experiences in a flash of time.

5.16 Near-Death Experiences

Some persons, most commonly those who had been involved in a life-threatening emergency or highly traumatic event, have reported experiencing a sense of detachment from their bodies and feelings of levitation at the time that they had been teetering between life and death. Though the initial reports of these so-called "NDEs" had initially been considered weak evidence of life outside the physical body, the growing number of them, which is now in the millions, and the consistency of them across diverse ethnic, cultural, and religious groups, is making them increasingly hard to dismiss. Further adding to their credibility is the fact that they are primarily unsolicited, unpaid, and apt to draw social scrutiny.

Nearly all persons who claim to have had an NDE say that their senses were sharpened and their awareness was expanded while divested of their physical bodies. Included among these are reports of blind persons being able to see and deaf persons being able to hear while detached from their physical bodies *(YouTube: Vicki Noratuk Blind Person NDE Accessed 4/12/19)*. Others claim to have watched themselves being resuscitated in the emergency room or operated on in the surgical suite despite being fully draped and deeply anesthetized. The detailed reports of such persons have been corroborated by the discovery of factual information that they could not have known had they been forced to rely on their physical senses[92,93].

In recognition of the importance of near-death studies to the field of medicine, an increasing number of physicians, scientists, and allied health professionals are joining the International Association for Near-Death Studies (IANDS). Today, IANDS conferences and meetings are being held at medical institutions around the world, and a growing number of scholarly articles and research findings related to NDEs are being published in prestigious medical and psychiatric journals.

In the largest study of its kind, Dr. Sam Parnia and his colleagues studied the outcomes of more than 2,000 patients who had undergone emergency resuscitation following cardiac arrest. The study, which involved fifteen medical centers in the United States, Europe, and Australia, found that among 330 survivors, 55 recalled having had some form of conscious awareness during the time that they were clinically dead, and nine of these individuals had NDEs. Among these, two recalled having been aware of the events that took place in the resuscitation area, one of whom provided information that was later corroborated by hospital staff that were present at the time[2].

Typically, there is a complete cessation of cortical activity (as indicated by an isoelectric flattening of the EEG) within less than a minute of cardiac arrest[94]. This despite the fact that neurons still have enough energy stores to maintain their membrane gradients and depolarize in a synchronized fashion[95]. Irreversible damage to the cerebrum does not occur for at least eight minutes after complete circulatory arrest[94]. Another peculiar observation is that a flattening of the EEG can sometimes precede circulatory arrest[96]. Even more inexplicably, a flattening of the EEG can sometimes be followed by a burst of synchronized electrical activity that equals or even exceeds that of the normal waking state[97,98]. Such phenomena would be hard to explain on a purely physiological basis. A more plausible explanation is that a pathological disruption of neurological function (or in some cases a willful choice of the individual) interrupts the dialogue between the mind and the brain. As a result, both the mind and the brain become increasingly quiescent, much as they do during the deeper stages of sleep[39].

If, beyond that point, there were enough will to live and enough return of neurological function to support a re-establishment of the normal dialogue between the mind and the brain, the person would regain corporeal consciousness. If not, the person would remain comatose until the mind were awoken by some extracorporeal influence. If the latter were to occur, the brain would again receive the mental input that, based on the concept of dualism, is believed to be the primary driver of synchronous neurological activity. Moreover, the resumption of neurological activity could potentially continue until the mind (together with the rest of the spiritual body) had passed outside the sphere of influence in accordance with Coulomb's Law[99]. This could explain the brief surge of synchronized neurological activity that is sometimes observed on end-of-life EEG tracings[97,98,100,101].

Because the mind, in the corporeal state, is theoretically buried deep within the brain, it must rely on the neurological system to receive input from the environment (Figure 12). By firing in distinct burst patterns, neurons hypothetically transfer the information to the mind in a language similar to Morse Code. In the world of electronics, this is known as "continuous wave modulation" and is the means by which television, radio, and cellular phone towers convey intelligible information to viewers and listeners. If any part of the neurological system were to break down, the associated input

TRANSFER OF INFORMATION FROM THE PHYSICAL BODY TO THE SPIRITUAL BODY

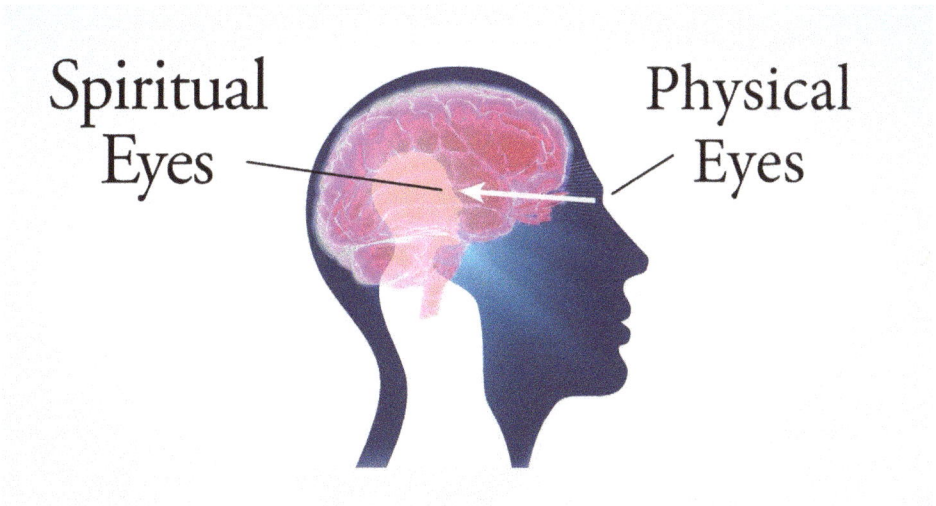

Figure 12. Schematic illustration of the relay of visual input from the physical eyes to the spiritual eyes via optic nerve tracts in the brain. © *Michael R. Binder, MD.*

would fail to reach the mind. This would explain the loss of sight when there is damage to the visual system, the loss of hearing when there is damage to the auditory system, etc... Note, however, that even if one or another sensory system were to become damaged, the mind could partially compensate by diverting the unused attentional energy to the sensory systems that remain functional. This idea is supported by a recent study in which persons who were either born blind or became blind at an early age were found to have a heightened sense of hearing, smell, and touch in comparison to subjects who were not blind[102]. Based on the results of numerous telephone and email telepathy studies, the mind also has the capacity to receive input without using the somatic sensory organs[103-106]. This was convincingly demonstrated by Grau et al.[107], who found that mentally-induced magnetic fields in the brain of one person could directly influence neurological activity in the brain of another person through a fully intact scalp. Because the associated magnetic fields must pass through the skin and skull before they can influence the mind, this mode of communication would be expected to be less discernible than normal communication. However, it can be more valuable because it involves a spontaneous transfer of thoughts and feelings and, thus, is less likely to be falsified.

In near-death and other out-of-body experiences, the mind theoretically leaves the thalamic cockpit and, like an ejected pilot, gains open access to all vibrational energy. What's more, it is able to process that energy consciously without having to rely on neurochemically-induced magnetic fields and the limitations of the slower-functioning brain. This would explain why the senses of NDErs become expanded, and their ability to receive and process information becomes amplified. The same reasoning would explain how blind persons are able to see and deaf persons are able to hear when they detach from their physical bodies *(Near-Death.com: People Born Blind Can See During NDE. Accessed 5/16/18)*. Then again, in a purely incorporeal state, the spiritual body would be devoid of sensory receptors for physical objects, thus explaining why NDErs generally report being unable to feel such objects (including the physical bodies of their loved ones) during an NDE despite being able to see them even more vividly than with their physical eyes *(YouTube: Kevin Zadai Died. What Jesus Showed Him Will Amaze You!).*

5.17 The Critical Divide Between Life and Death

The greatest mystery that the mind–brain duality helps solve is the subtle but critical distinction between life and death. From a medical standpoint, there is still no clear definition of when a person actually dies. The currently accepted definition, which defines death as a lack of responsiveness to nociceptive stimuli, a loss of brainstem reflexes, and a flattening of the EEG, is incompatible with the observation that these same biomarkers are intentionally (and reversibly) induced during general anesthesia[39]. Thus, these indicators are not adequately specific, nor are they able to define the exact moment of death. However, the idea that the mind is an energy body that is somehow connected to the physical body provides an anatomically–specific definition of death: death occurs when the mind (together with the rest of the spiritual body) separates from the physical body. This definition does not imply that all bodily functions come to a screeching halt the moment that the spiritual body separates from the physical body. Rather, it asserts that the spiritual body, which theoretically gives life to the physical body, stops driving bodily functions once it passes away from the physical body. That would explain why a flattening of the EEG, which suggests a weakening of the connection between the mind and brain (Figure 12), and a cessation of cardiac function, which suggests a loosening of the connection between the spiritual heart and the physical heart are soon, but not immediately, followed by a determination of death based on a cessation of bodily functions.

6.0 Concluding Comment

Despite modern advances in the understanding of brain structure and function, there are still many mental and neurological phenomena that remain unexplained from a psychophysiological standpoint. However, converging lines of clinical, anatomical, and biophysical evidence suggest that the human mind, rather than being a mere product of brain function, is a thinking, feeling, body of energy that is highly resonant with, but functionally distinct from, the brain. The proposed point of interface between the mind and the brain is the thalamus, the hub of virtually all information coming into the brain and the center of exchange for virtually all information processed by the brain. Dwelling within the thalamus is the human mind, seated like a pilot in the cockpit of an airplane. From this strategic position, the mind theoretically uses the TRN as a computer touchscreen through which it can control the brain and, by extension, the rest of the body via simple shifts in attention.

These new insights into the anatomy of the cognitive-emotional system provide simple answers to some of the most challenging questions in the fields of psychology, psychiatry, and neurology. Although some of the foregoing explanations may be difficult to prove scientifically, they would be far more difficult to disprove. Moreover, the utility, logic, and simplicity of the explanations are themselves evidence of their validity. Many of the greatest scientists, philosophers, and thinkers throughout history have said that the beauty and simplicity of a theory is greater evidence of truth than scientific experimentation. "Beauty brings with itself evidence that enlightens without mediation," wrote Hans Von Balthasar, one of history's most renowned philosophers.

It is my hope that these new insights, which echo the ideas of some of the greatest thinkers of the past, will be a springboard for renewed scientific investigation into the mind-brain duality of the cognitive-emotional system. Undoubtedly, a more comprehensive understanding of this foundational part of human anatomy would lead to a more comprehensive understanding of human psychophysiology, psychiatric disorders, and the critical divide between life and death. Even more important, it would reinforce the hope that life does not end with the death of the physical body.

+ + +

References

1. Moody RA. (1975). Life after life. Mockingbird Books.

2. Parnia S, Spearpoint K, de Vos G, Fenwick P, Goldberg D, Yang J, Zhu J, Baker K, Killingback H, McLean P, Wood M, Zafari AM, Dickert N, Beisteiner R, Sterz F, Berger M, Warlow C, Bullock S, Lovett S, McPara RMS, Marti-Navarette S, Cushing P, Wills P, Harris K, Sutton J, Walmsley A, Deakin CD, Little P, Farber M, Greyson B, Schoenfeld ER. (2014). AWARE—AWAreness during REsuscitation—A prospective study. Resuscitation. 85:1799-1805.

3. Penfield W. (1936). Epilepsy and surgical therapy. Archives of Neurology and Psychiatry. 36(3):449-484.

4. Boyden ES, Zang F, Bamberg E, Nagel G, Deisseroth K. (2005). Millisecond-timescale, genetically targeted optical control of neural activity. Nature Neuroscience. 8:1263-1268.

5. Al-Shargie, F, Kiguchi, M, Badruddin, N, Dass, SC, Hani, AFM, Tang, TB. (2016). Mental stress assessment using simultaneous measurement of EEG and fNIRS. Biomedical Optics Express. 7(10):3882-3898.

6. Binder MR. (2019-a). The multi-circuit neuronal hyperexcitability hypothesis of psychiatric disorders. American Journal of Clinical and Experimental Medicine. 7(1):12-30.

7. Binder MR. (2019-b). Electrophysiology of seizure disorders may hold key to the pathophysiology of psychiatric disorders. American Journal of Clinical and Experimental Medicine. 7(5):103-110.

8. Grunze HCR. (2008). The effectiveness of anticonvulsants in psychiatric disorders. Dialogues in Clinical Neuroscience. 10(1):77-89.

9. Fleming KC, Volcheck MM. (2015). Central Sensitization Syndrome and the initial evaluation of a patient with fibromyalgia: a review. Rambam Maimonides Medical Journal. 6(2):e0020.

10. McEwen BS. (2004). Protection and damage from acute and chronic stress: allostasis and allostatic overload and relevance to the pathophysiology of psychiatric disorders. Annals of the New York Academy of Sciences. 1032:1-7.

11. Lazarus RS. (1903). From psychological stress to the emotions: a history of changing outlooks. Annual Review of Psychology. 44:1-21.

12. Post RM. (2007). Kindling and sensitization as models for affective episode recurrence, cyclicity, and tolerance phenomena. Neuroscience & Biobehavioral Review. 31(6):858-873.

13. McKee HR, Privitera, MD. (2017). Stress as a seizure precipitant: identification, associated factors, and treatment options. Seizure. 44: 21-26.

14. McFadden J. Integrating information in the brain's EM field: the cemi field theory of consciousness. Neuroscience of Consciousness. 2020; 2020(1).

15. Pockett S. The electromagnetic field theory of consciousness: A testable hypothesis about the characteristics of conscious as opposed to non-conscious fields. Journal of Consciousness Studies. 2012; 19(11-12):191-223.

16. Xu Y, Jia Y, Ma J, Hayat T, Alsaedi A. (2018). Collective responses in electrical activities of neurons under field coupling. https://doi.org/10.1038/s41598-018-19858-1.

17. Crick F. (1984). Function of the thalamic reticular complex: The searchlight hypothesis. Proceedings of the National Academy of Sciences. 81:4586-4590.

18. Theyel BB, Llano AL, Sherman SM. (2010). The corticothalamocortical circuit drives higher-order cortex in the mouse. Nature Neuroscience. 13:84-88.

19. Baroncelli L, Braschi C, Spolidoro M, Begenisic T, Maffei L, Sale A. (2011). Brain plasticity and disease: a matter of inhibition. Neural Plasticity. 2011.

20. Herrero MT, Insausti R, Estrada C. (2015). Reference model in neuroscience and biobehavioral psychology. In: Brain mapping: An encyclopedic reference. Vol. 2: Anatomy and Physiology Systems: 219-242.

21. Min B-K. (2010). A thalamic reticular networking model of consciousness. Theoretical Biology and Medical Modelling. 7:10. http://dx.doi.org/10.1186/1742-4682-7-10.

22. Treisman A. (1977). Focused attention in the perception and retrieval of multidimensional stimuli. Perception & Psychophysics. 22(1):1-11.

23. Treisman A, Gelade GA. (1980). A feature integration theory of attention. Cognitive Psychology. 12:97-136.

24. Treisman A, Schmidt H. (1982). Illusory conjunctions in the perception of objects. Cognitive Psychology. 14:107-141.

25. Julesz B. (1980). Spacial nonlinearities in the instantaneous perception of textures with identical power spectra. Philosophical Transactions of the Royal Society of London B. 290:83-94.

26. Julesz B. (1981). Textons, the elements of texture perception, and their interactions. Nature. 290:91-97.

27. Bergen JR, Julesz B. (1983). Parallel versus serial processing in rapid pattern discrimination. Nature. 303:696-698.

28. Houser CR, Vaughn JE, Barber RP, Roberts E. (1980). GABA neurons are the major cell type of the nucleus reticularis thalami. Brain Research. 200:341-354.

29. Ohara PT, Lieberman AR, Hunt SP, Wu J-Y. (1983). Neural elements containing glutamic acid decarboxylase (GAD) in the dorsal lateral geniculate nucleus of the rat; immunohistochemical studies by light and electron microscopy. Neuroscience. 8(2):189-211.

30. Alkire MT, Hudetz AG, Tononi G. (2008). Consciousness and anesthesia. Science. 322(5903):876-880.

31. Kawkabani K. (2018). Preserved consciousness in the absence of a cerebral cortex, the legal and ethical implications of redefining consciousness and its neural correlates: A case for a subcortical system generating affective consciousness. Neuroscience and Neurobiology Commons, Honors Research Projects. 734.

32. Hindman J, Bowren MD, Bruss J, Wright B, Geerling JC, Boes AD. (2018). Thalamic strokes that severely impair arousal extend into the brainstem. Annals of Neurology. 84(6):926-930.

33. Posner JB, Plum F. (2007). Contemporary neurology series. 4. Oxford University Press; Oxford; New York: Plum and Posner's Diagnosis of Stupor and Coma; p. xiv.p. 401.

34. Schiff ND, Giacino JT, Kalmar K, Victor JD, Baker K. (2007). Behavioural improvements with thalamic stimulation after severe traumatic brain injury. Nature. 448(7153):600-603.

35. Lemaire J-J, Sontheimer A, Pereira B, Coste J, Rosenberg S, Sarret C, Coll G, Gabrillargues J, Jean B, Gillart T, Coste A, Roche B, Kelly A, Pontier B, Feschet F. (2018). Deep brain stimulation in five patients with severe disorders of consciousness. Annals of Clinical and Translational Neurology. 5(11):1372-1384.

36. Brown RE, Basheer R, McKenna JT, Strecker RE, McCarley RW. (2012). Control of sleep and wakefulness. Physiological Reviews. 92(3):1087-1187.

37. Singh C, Rihel J, Prober DA. (2017). Neuropeptide Y regulates sleep by modulating noradrenergic signaling. Current Biology. 27(24):3796-3811.e5.

38. Lee DA, Andreev A, Truong TV, Chen A, Hill AJ, Oikonomou G,and Pham U, Hong YK, Tran S, Glass L, Sapin V, Engle J, Fraser SE, Prober DA. (2017). Genetic and neuronal regulation of sleep by neuropeptide VF. eLife. 6 Art. No. e25727.

39. Brown EN, Lydic R, Schiff ND. (2010). General anesthesia, sleep, and coma. New England Journal of Medicine. 263(27):2638-2650.

40. Binder MR. (2019-c). Introducing the term "Neuroregulator" in psychiatry. American Journal of Clinical and Experimental Medicine. 7(3):66-70.

41. Casali AG, Gosseries O, Rosanova M, Boly M, Sarasso S, Casali KR, Casarotto S, Bruno M-A, Laureys S, Tononi G, Massimini M. (2013). A theoretically based index of consciousness independent of sensory processing and behavior. Science Translational Medicine. 5(198):198ra105.

42. Nakajima M, Halassa MM. (2017). Thalamic control of functional cortical connectivity. Current Opinion in Neurobiology. 44:127-131.

43. Merker B. (2007). Consciousness without a cerebral cortex: A challenge for neuroscience and medicine. Behavioral and Brain Sciences, 30(1): 63-134.

44. Llinás R, Jahnsen H. (1982). Electrophysiology of mammalian thalamic neurons in vitro. Nature (London). 297(5865):406-408.

45. Jahnsen H, Llinás R. (1984-a). Electrophysiological properties of guinea pig thalamic neurones: an in vitro study. Journal of Physiology. 349(1):205-226.

46. Jahnsen H, Llinás R. (1984-b). Ionic basis for the electro-responsiveness and oscillatory properties of guinea-pig thalamic neurons in vitro. Journal of Physiology. 349:227-247.

47. Portas CM, Rees G, Howseman AM, Josephs O, Turner R, Frith CD. (1998). A specific role for the thalamus in mediating the interaction of attention and arousal in humans. Journal of Neuroscience. 18(21):8979-8989.

48. Smith BD, Meyers M, Kline R, Bozman A. (1987). Hemispheric asymmetry and emotion: Lateralized parietal processing of affect and cognition. Biological Psychology. 25(3):247-260.

49. Goddard GV, McIntyre DC, Leech CK. (1969). A permanent change in brain function resulting from daily electrical stimulation. Experimental Neurology. 25:295-330.

50. Okeju O, Song AH, Hamilos AE, Pavone KJ, Flores FJ, Brown EN, Purdon PL. (2016). Electroencephalogram signatures of ketamine anesthesia-induced unconsciousness. Clinical Neurophysiology. 127(6):2414-2422.

51. Blumenfeld H. (2005). Consciousness and epilepsy: why are patients with absence seizures absent? Progress in Brain Research. 150:271-286.

52. Bragg EM, Fairless EA, Liu S, Briggs F. (2017). Morphology of visual sector thalamic reticular neurons in the macaque monkey suggests retinotopically specialized, parallel stream-mixed Input to the lateral geniculate nucleus. Journal of Comparative Neurology. 525(5):1273-1290.

53. Lübke J. (1993). *OnlineLibrary.wiley.com: Morphology of neurons in the thalamic reticular nucleus (TRN) of mammals as revealed by intracellular injections into fixed brain slices.* Journal of Comparative Neurology. 329(4).

54. Wang S, Tudusciuc O, Mamelak AN, Ross IB, Adolphs R, Rutishauser U. (2014). Neurons in the human amygdala selective for perceived emotion. Proceedings of the National Academy of Sciences. 111(30):E3110-E3119.

55. Jimenez JC, Su K, Goldberg AR, Luna VM, Biane JS, Ordek G, Zhou P, Ong SK, Wright MA, Zweifel L, Paninski L, Hen R, Kheirbek MA. (2018). Anxiety cells in a hippocampal-hypothalamic circuit. Neuron. 97(3):670-683.e6.

56. Wang S, Yu R, Tyszka JM, Zhen S, Kovach C, Sun S, Huang Y, Hurlemann R, Ross IB, Chung JM, Mamelak AN, Adophs R, Rutishauser U. (2017). The human amygdala parametrically encodes the intensity of specific facial emotions and their categorical ambiguity. Nature Communications. 8:14821.

57. Woolf CJ. (2011). Central sensitization: implications for the diagnosis and treatment of pain. Pain. 153(3 suppl): S2-15.

58. Melloni L, Molina C, Pena M, Torres D, Singer W, Rodriguez E. (2007). Synchronization of neural activity across cortical areas correlates with conscious perception. Journal of Neuroscience. 27(11):2858-2865.

59. Llinás R, Ribary U. (1993). Coherent 40-Hz oscillation characterizes dream state in humans. Proceedings of the National Academy of Sciences. 90(5):2078–2081.

60. Llinás RR, Paré D. (1991). Of dreaming and wakefulness. Neuroscience. 44(3):521-535.

61. Erlij D, Acosta-Garcia J, Rojas-Márquez M, González-Hernández B, Escartín-Perez E, Aceves J, Florán B. (2012). Dopamine D4 receptor stimulation in GABAergic projections of the globus pallidus to the reticular thalamic nucleus and the substantia nigra reticulata of the rat decreases locomotor activity. Neuropharmacology. 62(2):1111-1118.

62. Rasia-Filho AA, Londero RG, Achaval M. (2000). Functional activities of the amygdala: an overview. Journal of Psychiatry and Neuroscience. 25(1):14-23.

63. Johnstone T, van Reekum CM, Urry HL, Kalin NH, Davidson, RJ. (2007). Failure to regulate: counterproductive recruitment of top-down prefrontal-subcortical circuitry in major depression. Journal of Neuroscience. 27(33):8877-8884.

64. Leuchter AF, Cook IA, Hunter AM, Cai C, Horvath S. (2012). Resting- state quantitative electroencephalography reveals increased neurophysiologic connectivity in depression. PloS One. 7(2):1-13. e32508.

65. Ferreira MAR, O'Donovan MC, Meng YA, Jones IR, Ruderfer DM, Jones L, Fan J, Kirov G, Perlis RH, Green EK, Smoller JW, Grozeva D, Stone J, Nikolov I, Chambert K, Hamshere ML, Nimgaonkar VL, Moskvina V, Thase ME, Caesar S, Sachs GS, Franklin J, Gordon-Smith K, Ardlie KG, Gabriel SB, Fraser C,

Blumenstiel B, Defelice M, Breen G, Gill M, Morris DW, Elkin A, Muir WJ, McGhee KA, Williamson R, MacIntyre DJ, MacLean AW, St. Clair D, Robinson M, Van Beck M, Pereira ACP, Kandaswamy R, McQuillin A, Collier, DA, Bass NJ, Young AH, Lawrence J, Ferrier IN, Anjorin A, Farmer A, Curtis D, Scolnick EM, McGuffin P, Daly MJ, Corvin AP, Holmans PA, Blackwood DH, Wellcome Trust Case Control Consortium, Gurling HM, Owen MJ, Purcell SM, Sklar P, Craddock N. (2008). Collaborative genome-wide association analysis supports a role for ANK3 and CACNA1C in bipolar disorder. Nature Genetics. 40(9):1056–1058.

66. Yuan A, Yi Z, Wang Q, Sun J, Li Z, Du Y, Zhang C, Yu T, Fan J, Li H, Yu S. (2012). ANK3 as a risk gene for schizophrenia: new data in Han Chinese and meta analysis. American Journal of Medical Genetics Part B: Journal of Neuropsychiatric Genetics. 159B(8):997–1005.

67. Lopez AY, Wang X, Xu M, Maheshwari A, Curry D, Lam S, Adesina AM, Noebels JL, Sun Q-Q, Cooper, EC. (2017). Ankyrin-G isoform imbalance and interneuronopathy link epilepsy and bipolar disorder. Molecular Psychiatry. 22(10):1464–1472.

68. Green EK, Grozeva D, Jones I, Jones L, Kirov G, Caesar S, Gordon-Smith K, Fraser C, Forty L, Russell E, Hamshere ML, Moskvina V, Nikolov I, Farmer A, McGuffin P, Wellcome Trust Case Control Consortium, Holmans PA, Owen MJ, O'Donovan MC, Craddock N. (2010) The bipolar disorder risk allele at CACNA1C also confers risk of recurrent major depression and of schizophrenia. Molecular Psychiatry. 15(10):1016–1022.

69. Liu Y, Blackwood DH, Caesar S, de Geus EJ, Farmer A, Ferreira MA, Ferrier IN, Fraser C, Gordon-Smith K, Green EK, Grozeva D, Gurling HM, Hamshere ML, Heutink P, Holmans PA, Hoogendijk WJ, Jan Hottenga J, Jones L, Jones IR, Kirov G, Lin D, McGuffin P, Moskvina V, Nolen WA, Perlis RH, Posthuma D, Scolnick EM, Smit AB, Smit JH, Smoller JW, St. Clair D, van Dyck R, Verhage M, Wellcome Trust Case-Control Consortium, Willemsen G, Young AH, Zandbelt T, Boomsma DI, Craddock N, O'Donovan MC, Owen MJ, Penninx BWJH, Purcell S, Sklar P, Sullivan PF. (2011) Meta-analysis of genome-wide association data of bipolar disorder and major depressive disorder. Molecular Psychiatry. 16(1).

70. Iqbal Z, Vandeweyer G, van der Voet M, Waryah AM; Zahoor MY, Besseling JA, Roca LT, Vulto-van S, Anneke T, Nijhof B, Kramer JM, Van der Aa N, Ansar M; Peeters H, Helsmoortel C, Gilissen C, Vissers L, Veltman JA, de Brouwer APM,

Kooy RF; Riazuddin S, Schenck A, van Bokhoven H, Rooms L. (2013) Homozygous and heterozygous disruptions of ANK3: at the crossroads of neurodevelopmental and psychiatric disorders. Human Molecular Genetics. 22:1960–1970.

71. Subramanian J, Dye L, Morozov, A. (2013). Rap1 signaling prevents L-type calcium channel-dependent neurotransmitter release. Journal of Neuroscience. 33(17):7245-7252.

72. Santos M, D'Amico D, Spadoni O, Amador-Arjona A, Stork O, Dierssen M. (2013). Hippocampal hyperexcitability underlies enhanced fear memories in TgNTRK3, a panic disorder mouse model. Journal of Neuroscience. 33(38):15259-15271.

73. Contractor A, Klyachko VA, Portera-Cailliau C. (2015). Altered neuronal and circuit excitability in fragile X syndrome. Neuron. 87(4):699-715.

74. O'Brien NL, Way MJ, Kandaswamy R, Fiorentino A, Sharp SI, Quadri G, Alex J, Anjorin A, Ball D, Cherian R, Dar K, Gormez A, Guerrini I, Heydtmann M, Hillman A, Lankappa S, Lydall G, O'Kane A, Patel S, Quested D, Smith I, Thomson AD, Bass NJ, Morgan MY, Curtis D, McQuillin A. (2014). The functional GRM3 Kozak sequence variant rs148754219 affects the risk of schizophrenia and alcohol dependence as well as bipolar disorder. Psychiatric Genetics. 24:277–278.

75. Schizophrenia Working Group of the Psychiatric Genomics Consortium: Ripke S, Neale BM, [...], O'Donovan MC. (2014). Biological insights from 108 schizophrenia-associated genetic loci. Nature. 511(7510):421-427.

76. Freedman R, Coon H, Myles-Worsley M, Orr-Urtreger A, Olincy A, Davis A, Polymeropoulos M, Holik J, Hopkins J, Hoff M, Rosenthal J, Waldo MC, Reimherr F, Wender P, Yaw J, Young DA, Breese CR, Adams C, Patterson D, Adler LE, Kruglyak L, Leonard S, Byerley W. (1997). Linkage of a neurophysiological deficit in schizophrenia to a chromosome 15 locus. Proceedings of the National Academy of Sciences. 94(2):587–592.

77. Pizzarelli R, Cherubini E. (2011). Alterations of GABAergic signaling in autism spectrum disorders. Neural Plasticity. 1011:157193.

78. Cassidy CM, Balsam PE, Weinstein JJ. (2018). A perceptual inference mechanism for hallucinations linked to striatal dopamine. Current Biology. 28:4. (Accessed 9/28/18).

79. Gittelman JX, Perke DJ, Portfors CV. (2013). Dopamine modulates auditory responses in the inferior colliculus in a heterogeneous manner. Journal of the Association for Research in Otolaryngology. 14(5):719-29.

80. Ford JM, Mathalon DH, Kalba S, Whitfield S, Faustman WO, Roth WT. (2001). Cortical responsiveness during talking and listening in schizophrenia: an event-related brain potential study. Biological Psychiatry. 50(7):540-549.

81. Carhart-Harris RL, Erritzoe D, Williams T, Stone JM, Reed, LJ, Colasanti A, Tyacke RJ, Leech R, Malizia AL, Murphy K, Hobden P, Evans J, Feilding A, Wise RG, Nutt DJ. (2012). Neural correlates of the psychedelic state as determined by fMRI studies with psilocybin. Proceedings of the National Academy of Sciences. 109(6):2138-2143.

82. Braun A. (1997). Regional cerebral blood flow throughout the sleep-wake cycle. An H2(15)O PET study. Brain. 120(7):1173–1197.

83. Siclari F, Baird B, Perogamvros L, Bernardi G, LaRocque JJ, Riedner B, Boly M, Postle BR, Tononi G. (2017). The neural correlates of dreaming. Nature Neuroscience. 20(6):872–878.

84. Solms M. (2014). The neuropsychology of dreams: a clinico-anatomical study (1 ed.). Psychology Press. ISBN: 978-1315806440.

85. De Ridder D, Elgoyhen AB, Romo R, Langguth B. (2011). Phantom percepts: tinnitus and pain as persisting aversive memory networks. Proceedings of the National Academy of Sciences. 108(20):8075–8080

86. Nyström B, Hagbarth K-E. (1981). Microelectrode recordings from transected nerves in amputees with phantom limb pain. Neuroscience Letters. 27(2):211-216.

87. Mercier C, Sirigu A. (2009). Training with virtual visual feedback to alleviate phantom limb pain. Neurorehabilitation & Neural Repair. 23(6):587-594.

88. Courchesne E, Mouton PR, Calhoun ME, Semendeferi K, Ahrens-Barbeau C, Hallet MJ, Barnes CC, Pierce K. (2011) Neuron number and size in prefrontal cortex of children with autism. Journal of the American Medical Association. 306(18):2001-2010.

89. Rane P, Cochran D, Hodge SM, Haselgrove C, Kennedy DN, Frazier JA. (2015). Connectivity in autism: A review of MRI connectivity studies. Harvard Review of Psychiatry. 23(4):223-244.

90. Schneider M. (1961). Survival and revival of the brain in anoxia and ischemia. In: Cerebral Anoxia and the Electroencephalogram. Pages 134-143. Edited by Gestaut H, Meyer JS. Thomas: Springfield, Illinois.

91. Brooks SJ, Savov V, Allzén E, Benedict C, Fredriksson R, Schioth HB. (2012). Exposure to subliminal arousing stimuli induces robust activation in the amygdala, hippocampus, anterior cingulate, insular cortex and primary visual cortex: a systematic meta-analysis of fMRI studies. NeuroImage. 59(3):2962–2973.

92. Alexander E. (2012). Proof of heaven: a neurosurgeon's journey into the afterlife. Simon and Schuster. New York, NY 10020.

93. Burke J. (2015). Imagine Heaven: near-death experiences, God's promises, and the exhilarating future that awaits you. Baker Books, Grand Rapids, MI.

94. Dreier JP, Major S, Foreman B, Winkler MKL, Kang EJ, Milakara D, Lemale CL, DiNapoli V, Hinzman JM, Woitzik J, Andaluz N, Carlson A, Hartings JA. (2018). Terminal spreading depolarization and electrical silence in death of human cerebral cortex. Annals of Neurology. 83(2):295-310.

95. Snyder A. (2009). Explaining and inducing savant skills: privileged access to lower level, less-processed information. Philosophical Transactions of the Royal Society of London. Series B, Biological Sciences. 364(1522):1399–1405.

96. Norton L, Gibson RM, Gofton T, Benson C. (2017). Electroencephalographic recordings during withdrawal of life-sustaining therapy until 30 minutes after declaration of death. Canadian Journal of Neurological Sciences. 44(2):139-145.

97. Chawla L, Seneff MG. (2013). End of life electrical surges. Proceedings of the National Academy of Sciences. 110(44)E4123.

98. Borjigin J, Lee U, Liu T, Pal D, Huff S, Klarr D, Sloboda J, Hernandez J, Wang MM, Mashour GA. (2013). Surge of neurophysiological coherence and connectivity in the dying brain. Proceedings of the National Academy of Sciences. 110(35):14432-14437.

99. Xu Y, Jia Y, Ma J, Hayat T, Alsaedi A. (2018). Collective responses in electrical activities of neurons under field coupling. https://doi.org/10.1038/s41598-018-19858-1.

100. Auyong DB, Klein SM, Gan TJ, Roche, AM, Olson DW, Habib AS. (2010). Processed electroencephalogram during donation after cardiac death. Anesthesia & Analgesia. 110(5):1428-1432.

101. van Rijn CM, Krijnen H, Menting-Hermeling S, Coenen AML. (2011). Decapitation in rats: Latency to unconsciousness and the 'wave of death.' PLoS ONE 6(1):e16514.

102. Bauer CM, Hirsch GV, Zajac L, Koo B-B, Collignon O, Merabet LB. (2017). Multimodal MR-imaging reveals large-scale structural and functional connectivity changes in profound early blindness. PlosOne. https://doi.org/10.1371/journal.pone.0173064.

103. Sheldrake R, Lambert M. (2007). An automated online telepathy test. Journal of Scientific Exploration. 21:511-522.

104. Sheldrake R, Smart P. (2003-a). Videotaped experiments on telephone telepathy. Journal of Parapsychology. 67:187-206.

105. Sheldrake R, Smart P. (2003-b). Experimental tests for telephone telepathy. Journal of the Society for Psychical Research. 67:184-199.

106. Sheldrake R, Smart P. (2005). Testing for telepathy in connection with emails. Perceptual and Motor Skills. 101:771-786.

107. Grau C, Ginhoux R, Riera A, Nguyen TL, Chauvat H, Berg M, Amengual JL, Pascual-Leone A, Ruffini G. (2014). PlosOne. *Journals.plos.org Conscious brain-to-brain communication in humans using non-Invasive technologies.*

ARTICLE 2

Does the Mysterious "Wave of Death" Mark the Critical Divide Between Life and Death?

Abstract: In both humans and animals, a peculiar spike on the electroencephalogram (EEG) during the dying process has been reported by several research groups. Some are touting it to be a neurophysiological explanation for the puzzling phenomenon of near-death experiences (NDEs). Based on the available clinical and electrophysiological evidence, this analysis contends that the so-called "wave of death" is not the cause of NDEs but rather evidence of them as the mind, upon separating from the brain during the transition from life to death, awakens to life outside the physical body and, in the process, drives a surge of neurological activity until it passes outside the area in which its magnetic field can induce neuronal discharges. To my knowledge, this is the first anatomically, psychophysiologically, and electromagnetically-based explanation that links end-of-life EEG activity to NDEs without discounting the seeming extracorporeal nature of those experiences. If this theory is correct, then end-of-life EEG tracings could be an objective marker for the transition from life to death. The identification of such a marker would have important practical implications with regard to the definition of death and the timing of the pronouncement of death in clinical practice.

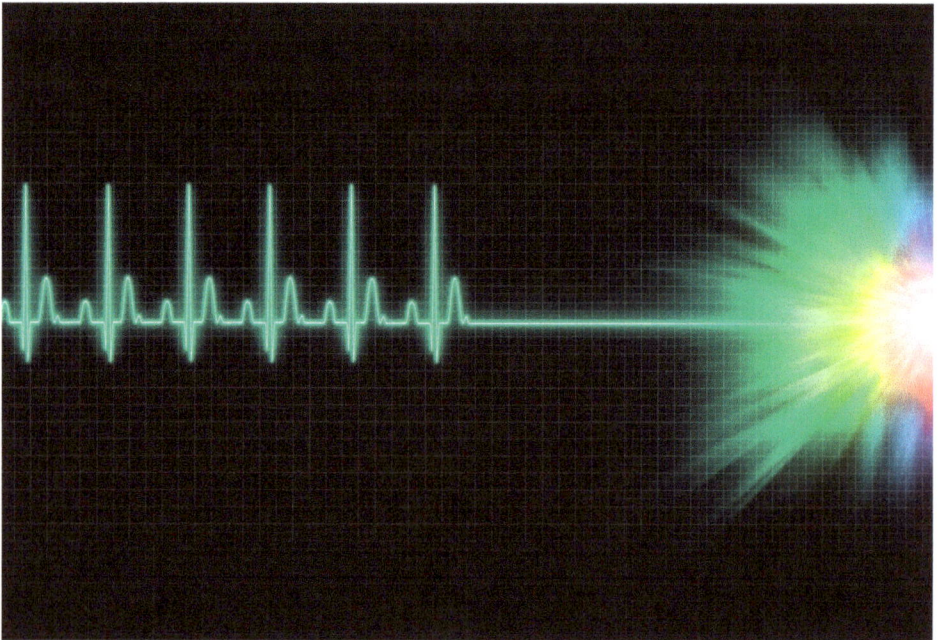

Introduction

Though death may in some cases be inevitable, there are important spiritual, religious, and existential questions that arise when a loved one is in a deeply unconscious state with diminishing hopes of recovery. There may also be disagreement, even among members of the healthcare team, about whether a gravely ill patient on advanced life support has any hope of survival or, in some cases, whether the patient is already dead. The matter is further complicated by the growing number of so-called "near-death experiences" (NDEs), in which persons who appear to have died on clinical grounds unexpectedly regain consciousness and, in some cases, make a full recovery. A better understanding of what happens during the transition from life to death and, correspondingly, a more reliable definition of death could help avoid a premature pronouncement of death and, conversely, an unnecessary prolongation of a process that is both labor-intensive and highly stressful for everyone involved.

A series of recent studies appears to have provided a clue to when a person dies. In both humans and animals, a brief spike in neurological activity has been identified after a near complete cessation of brainwave activity during the transition from life to death[1-4]. Specifically, the electroencephalogram (EEG) nearly flatlines, then spikes for a brief period (ranging from about 30 seconds to 30 minutes), before giving way to a multi-focal spreading wave of depolarization that initiates a plethora of toxic changes that end in irreversible cell injury[3,5].

In animals, total ischemia causes the EEG to flatline in just 20-30 seconds[5,6]. This cerebral silencing, which involves a hyperpolarization of neurons, is known as "non-spreading depression"[5]. During this phase of the response to hypoxia, there are still enough adenosine triphosphate (ATP) to maintain the ionic gradients that allow synchronized cellular messaging to occur[5]. That raises the question of why the EEG flattens at this time. It has been hypothesized that the shut down in neural signaling is a systems effort to conserve energy before the ATP pool is depleted[5].

However, a physiological mechanism for such a conservation process is lacking, and a similar flattening of the EEG has, in some cases, been observed in advance of cardiovascular arrest[7]. This raises the possibility that brainwave activity could be driven by something more than just pacemaker cells and weighted synaptic inputs. It reinvokes the idea that the mind could be a separate entity from the brain and that the process of "thinking" could involve a dialogue between the mind and the brain (Figure 1). If this were true, then any disruption in the mind–brain dialogue could cause a person to lapse into a coma.

DIALOGUE BETWEEN THE MIND AND THE BRAIN

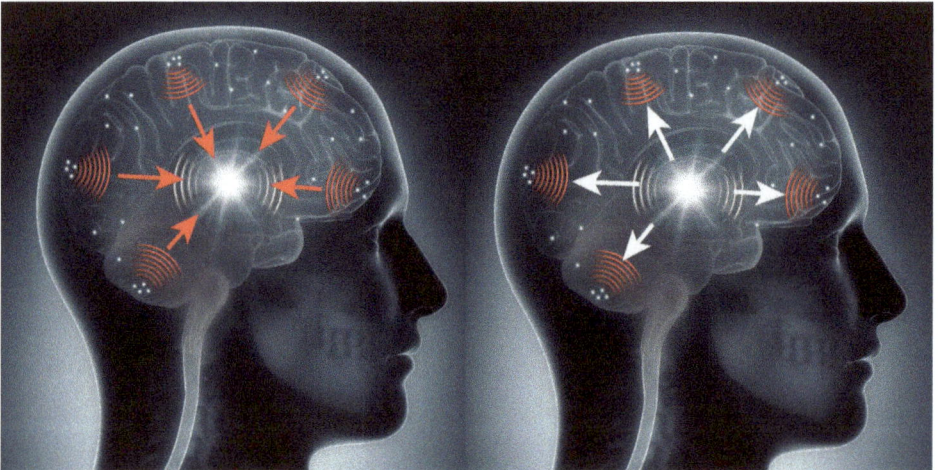

Figure 1. Schematic illustration of neurological input being relayed from the brain to the mind (above left), and mental output being relayed from the mind to the brain (above right). © *Michael R. Binder, MD.*

One of history's strongest proponents of the mind–brain duality was the pioneer in mathematics, science, and metaphysics René Descartes. Descartes believed not only that the mind was substantively different than the brain but also that it could function independent of the brain. However, his treatise on dualism was hampered by the mind–body problem: how could the mind and the brain communicate if their natures were different? A possible answer to that historic question arises from modern advances in chemistry, biology, and physics.

It is self-evident that mental processes involve energy. Mental effort is something that all of us are familiar with and exert every day. It follows then that mental effort, being a form of energy, could induce magnetic fields. These magnetic fields, in turn, could theoretically induce waves of depolarization in neurons that are uniquely responsive to those magnetic fields[8-11] (Figure 2). The reverse process could also occur[12], thus allowing the mind and the brain to communicate in the same language—electromagnetic energy. The idea that the mind is an independent, self-governing entity that works closely with the

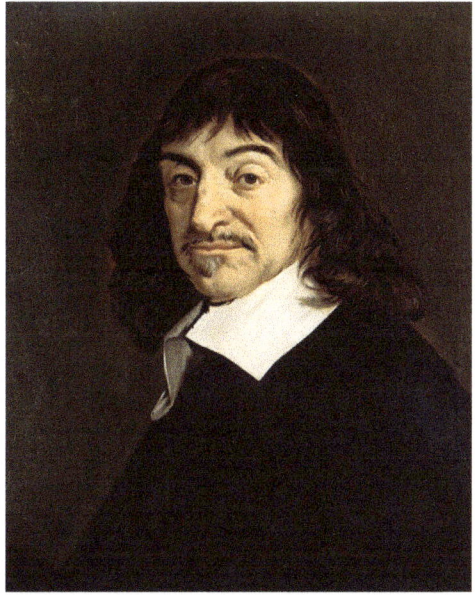

René Descartes (1596 – 1650)
French philosopher, mathematician, and scientist

brain could help explain many phenomena in psychology and psychiatry, including creative thought, self-discipline, stress-induced kindling of the brain, dream sleep (during which the mind is highly active yet partially disengaged from brain function)[13-15], and the onset of coma ahead of any significant depletion of ATP reserves or loss of ionic gradients.

Yet the most compelling evidence that the mind is an entity distinct from the brain comes from the growing number of NDEs, in which persons who have been on the brink of death due to a severe illness or injury claim to have separated from their bodies and had vivid experiences while in a comatose state[16,17]. Beyond the fact that these experiences, by definition, occur when the patient is either clinically dead or very close to death, the profound nature of them, the consistency of the descriptions across diverse cultural groups, and the fact that some of them include verifiable information is compelling evidence that they are something other than products of neurological activity.

INDUCTION OF MAGNETIC FIELDS BY NEUROLOGICAL ACTIVITY

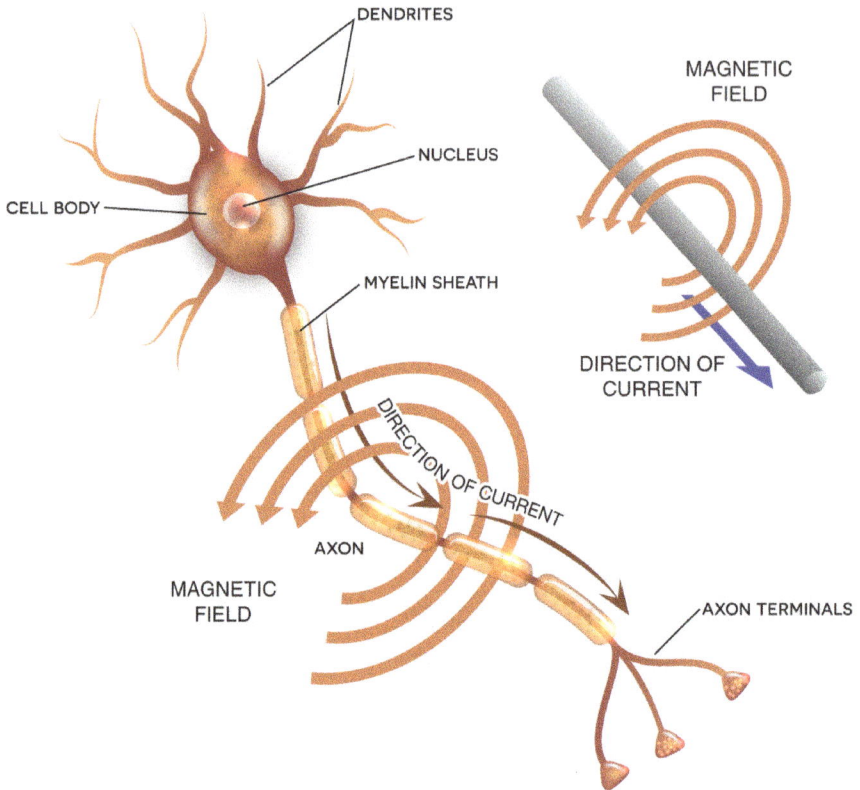

Figure 2. Schematic illustration of magnetic field induction via the electrochemical activity of neurons. © *Michael R. Binder, MD.*

From the perspective of a mind–brain duality of the cognitive–emotional system, any disruption of neurological function, such as that caused by ischemia or injury, would be expected to disrupt communications between the mind and the brain. As a result, both the mind and the brain would theoretically become increasingly quiescent. This idea is supported by the observation that deep sleep is associated with a slowing of the EEG that is virtually indistinguishable from that of the comatose state[18]. If there were enough will to live and enough return of neurological function to support the re-establishment of the normal dialogue between the mind and the brain, the person could presumably regain consciousness. If not, the person could be expected to either remain comatose or begin to separate from the brain and body.

Evidence of this comes from the unexpected association between the EEG tracing in the initial hours post cardiac arrest and the prognosis for survival in resuscitated patients. Lemmi et al.[19] found that regardless of the health of the brain either preceding or following cardiac arrest, the preservation of consciousness (or rapid regaining of it) was a strong predictor of survival, whereas those patients who were unconscious from the onset of cardiac arrest and remained unconscious until the time of their first EEG several hours later never left the hospital. Those patients who expressed an alpha rhythm intermixed with diffuse slowing were found to have intermediate chances of survival. These findings were corroborated by Westhall[20], who has studied the prognostic value of EEGs more extensively.

What may happen when there is a pathological loss of consciousness is that the brain, due to a disruption of thalamo-cortical function[21], stops stimulating the mind. This would presumably cause the mind to fall asleep, the result of which would be a cessation of the dialogue between the mind and the brain. Clinically, this would be consistent with the state known as "coma." What distinguishes this form of sleep from normal sleep is that it is initiated and perpetuated by a disruption of normal brain function; hence the lack of sleep-wake cycles, dream sleep, or responsiveness to pain. The greater the disruption of neurological function and the longer it persists, the smaller the chances that the brain will ever again be able to signal the mind to reawaken as it normally would from sleep. The mere fact that the mind-brain dialogue is being pathologically disrupted increases the risk that the mind will separate from the brain, as suggested by the fact that nearly half of all anesthesia-related deaths occur at therapeutic anesthetic doses[22]. This could help explain why those patients in the Lemmi study who remained conscious (or only briefly lost consciousness) during cardiac arrest had a better prognosis than those patients who lost consciousness and subsequently remained unconscious after being resuscitated.

Another important factor is the attitude of the patient. It has been said that the "spiritual body," of which the mind is the head, leaves the physical body when it becomes convinced that there is no longer any hope of survival or, in some cases, when it refuses to go on living. This is something that all human beings seem to know instinctively. For example, if a person were to suddenly lose consciousness due to an acute illness or severe injury, most bystanders would instinctively try to rouse the person back to consciousness. This is not always in vain, as there have been many instances in which such efforts were successful and may have even saved the person's life. From the perspective of the mind-brain duality of the cognitive-emotional system, such interventions as saying the person's name, touching the person's face, and holding the person's hand send messages to the mind via the somatosensory system, thus providing the neurological input that helps reestablish the dialogue between the mind and the brain. In the absence of these efforts, the unconscious person might begin to separate from the body, awaken to life outside the physical body (as presumably occurs in NDEs), and decide to leave the body permanently. Even in the absence of a life-threatening illness or injury, an intense desire to leave the world or flee from a dangerous situation could be enough to cause the spirit to dissociate from the body, thus explaining why the phenomenon of dissociation is most often precipitated by a highly traumatic or life-threatening event. In rare instances, fear can be so intense that it can theoretically drive an immediate and permanent separation between the mind and the body; hence the expression "scared to death."

Referring again to the importance of attitude, an acceptance of death is more likely to be assumed by the patient with multiple debilitating medical problems than by the patient who is otherwise in good health. This could help explain the observed difference in neurological response to hypoxia in those patients who have a positive outlook toward recovery in comparison to those who have a negative outlook. For example, when a bolus of short-acting adenosine is used to temporarily stop the heart in patients undergoing thoracic aorta endovascular repair, EEG power is reduced to 57% but returns to normal with 5 minutes of cardiac arrest[23]. This is in contrast to patients who, after unexpectedly experiencing a cardiac arrest, typically fail to make such a quick recovery even if, once resuscitated, their brains are just as adequately reoxygenated as those who undergo elective endovascular repairs. Of course, it could be argued that such patients are more severely ill than their surgical counterparts. However, in most cases, their illnesses involve the heart, not the brain. Hence, the observed difference in neurological response would be difficult to explain on a purely physiological basis. A more likely explanation is that the two groups differ in their degree of hope. In general, one would expect the patient who is undergoing an elective surgical procedure in anticipation of making a full recovery to have more hope than the patient who is unexpectedly experiencing a life-threatening cardiac arrest. Hope causes one to embrace life and, thus, more tightly engage the body, whereas a lack thereof reduces one's affinity for life and for the body. This is exemplified by the observation that manic patients have little interest in sleep, whereas depressed patients tend to oversleep despite the fact that their brain's, like those of manic patients, have difficulty shutting off[24-26]. The same reasoning could be applied to the dying patient, thus helping to explain why a person who has more hope and a greater desire to live is generally more likely to emerge from a comatose state than a person who has less hope and a lesser desire to live.

These ideas also appear to be supported by animal studies. In an effort to determine whether decapitation is a humane method of euthanasia in awake laboratory animals, van Rijn et al.[1] monitored the EEGs of seven rats before and after decapitation via guillotine. When fully conscious rats were decapitated, EEG power in the 13-100 Hz range fell to one-half after just 4 seconds, indicating that, at that point, the animals were too deeply unconscious to experience pain or perceive stimuli (Figure 3, Graph a). The EEG proceeded to flatline after another 11 seconds. This is hardly enough time for hypoxia to have had such a profound effect on brain function since there would still have been enough ATP to maintain the ionic gradients that are necessary for the production of action potentials and related cellular processes[27]. A more plausible explanation is that once decapitated, the rats lost consciousness awareness for a brief period of time, and then, as they began to separate from their dying bodies, regained consciousness—not corporeal consciousness but incorporeal consciousness. That the rats had regained awareness, though seemingly unconscious, is suggested by the surge of *synchronized* neurological activity that was consistently observed approximately 50 seconds post-decapitation (Figure 3, Graph b) . Of course, one could argue that this neurological activity could have been purely physiological, but that would fail to explain the high coherence of the activity, which was consistent with normal conscious processing. It would also fail to recognize the significance of the similarity in both the timing and duration of the same phenomenon that in humans has been linked to known conscious experiences; that is, NDEs. Hence, the electrical surge in these animals more likely reflects a reawakening of the mind as it begins to separate from the brain. Based on Coulomb's Law, which states that the intensity of a magnetic field is inversely proportional to the distance from its source, the mind of a dying mouse could, at least for a brief time, remain in close enough proximity to the brain to influence it before it passes away from it. Interestingly, a comparable group of rats that had been anesthetized prior to decapitation showed the same decline in EEG power; however, the death wave was significantly delayed, beginning after approximately 80 seconds in comparison to just 50 seconds in the conscious rats (Figure 3, Graph b). The additional 30-second delay in the anesthetized rats could reflect the temporary interference that anesthesia would have had in the animal's ability to recognize that something catastrophic had happened, something that was clearly incompatible with life. Hence the delay in the animal's willingness to surrender its life.

In a similar study, Borjigin et al.[2] performed continuous EEG monitoring in two groups of rats, one undergoing experimentally-induced cardiac arrest in a waking state, and the other in an anesthetized state. As in the van Rijn study, the investigators identified a transient surge of electrical activity just prior to death. More specifically, these were global, highly coherent, synchronous gamma oscillations that exhibited tight phase-coupling to both theta and alpha band frequencies in conjunction with an eightfold increase in anterior–posterior-directed connectivity (normally associated with conscious processing) and a fivefold increase in bottom-up information flow (normally associated with sensory processing)[2,28]. This high frequency neurological activity exceeded the levels found during the conscious waking state, demonstrating to the authors that the brain can generate neural correlates of consciousness (and even heightened awareness) during the transition from life to death. The so-called "wave of death" was also observed when carbon dioxide inhalation

EEG IN DEATH BY DECAPITATION IN RATS

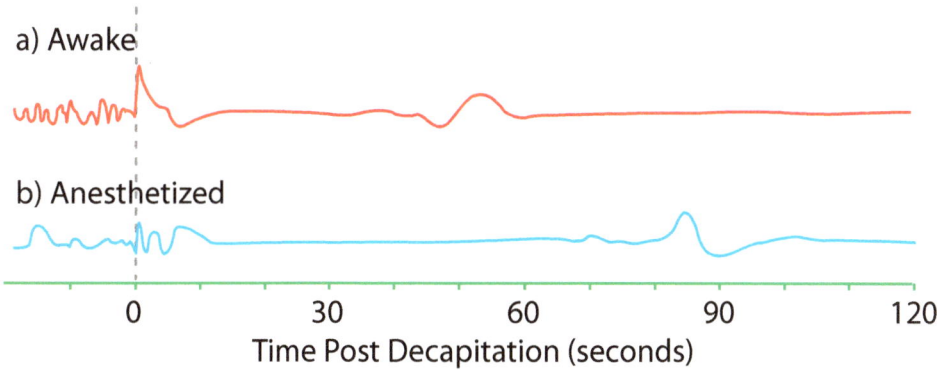

a) Awake

b) Anesthetized

Time Post Decapitation (seconds)

Figure 3. Electroencephalograms of (a) waking rats pre and post-decapitation; (b) anesthetized rats pre and post-decapitation. Adapted from van Rijn CM, et al. Decapitation in rats: Latency to unconsciousness and the 'wave of death'[1].

was used as an alternative form of death, thus demonstrating that the surge of brainwave activity was not uniquely related to death by cardiac arrest[2]. In these experiments, one would not expect there to have been any group differences in the timing of the death wave because cardiac arrest, which in animals causes a loss of consciousness before there is any clear recognition of trauma or disability, is not as indicative of impending death as decapitation. Accordingly, these experiments did not show any group differences in the timing of the wave of death.

In an effort to monitor changes in the level of consciousness during the dying process in humans, Chawla and Seneff[3] used an integer-based system to precisely monitor blood pressure in relation to level of alertness, as measured by muscle and frontal activity, in a series of seven patients who were neurologically intact before a decision was made, based on severity of illness, to withdraw life support. In each case, a loss of blood pressure, as measured by an indwelling arterial line, was followed by the expected loss of muscle tone and EEG activity. However, this was followed by a transient surge in EEG activity that, as observed in the mouse study, approached levels normally associated with consciousness. Consciousness in this context could more aptly be referred to as "corporeal consciousness" because it is mediated by the brain. This is in contrast to "incorporeal conscious," which is theoretically independent of the brain and body. In each case, the spike was of short duration (30–180 seconds) and was followed by a decline in activity to a level associated with burst suppression. The investigators were able to confirm that this activity was not due to artifact and that, on the contrary, it was a high-frequency wave form that could realistically explain the vivid, organized mental experiences reported by NDErs. The authors reported that they had observed these EEG spikes (which were generally of higher frequency than those observed in animals) in more than 20 other patients immediately prior to the pronouncement of death. They also pointed out, however, that they had observed these spikes in only about half of the patients who had expired in the intensive care unit[3]. This last observation would be difficult to explain if the wave of death were merely a normal correlate of neurological deterioration.

In another report, Auyong et al.[4] had been using the same integer-based system to monitor cognitive function during the process of "organ donation after cardiac death" in a patient who was irreversibly brain-damaged but technically not brain-dead. The patient was unresponsive to stimulation and exhibited flaccid paralysis on physical examination. The patient's bispectral index (BIS) scores, which reflect level of consciousness, ranged from 1 to 20 until a few minutes after life support was discontinued, at which point the BIS (in the absence of any electromyographic interference on the monitor) rapidly rose to 92 (Figure 4). The BIS values continued to range between 85 and 95 for approximately 23 minutes, and then abruptly fell to less than 4. This apparent movement to a lighter plane of anesthesia would be difficult to explain on a purely physiological basis not only because the patient was irreversibly brain-damaged but also because the collapse of cerebral circulation following the discontinuation of life support would have further impaired brain function. Yet the brain expressed a burst of synchronized, coherent, bi-frontal oscillations, signals that are the electrophysiological signature of normal conscious processing. The same phenomenon, which had a duration of 3–4 minutes, was observed in two other patients, both of whom were free of hypnotic or anesthetic drugs and in whom there were no significant changes in monitoring artifact.

What may have happened in these cases is that the mind regained conscious awareness—not corporeal awareness but incorporeal awareness—either by spontaneously disengaging from the malfunctioning brain or by being drawn away from it by some outside influence. In theory, this reawakening would be similar to being awoken by morning sunlight inasmuch as sleep is brought about by a loss of sensory input, and, conversely, awakening is brought about by a return of sensory input. In the Auyong study, a loss of sensory input was caused by the malfunctioning brain, and a return of sensory input theoretically

WAVE OF DEATH IN HUMANS

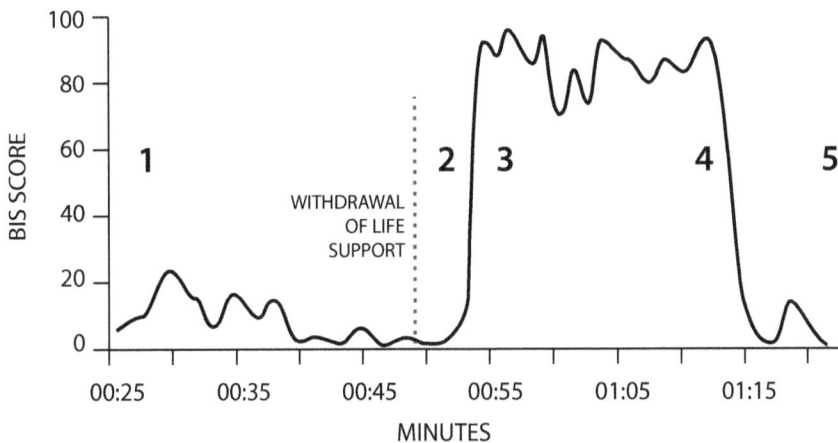

Figure 4. Conceptual reconstruction of real-time electroencephalographic data from an irreversibly brain-damaged (but not brain-dead) comatose patient pre and post-removal of life support in preparation for organ donation surgery. Prior to the removal of life support, BIS scores ranged between 1 and 20 (points 1-2 on the graph). Within 5 minutes of withdrawing life support, the BIS value abruptly increased from 1 to 92 (point 3) without evidence of EMG interference on the BIS monitor. Heart rate and oxygen saturation remained high for the first 8 minutes after withdrawal of care. 25 minutes after the withdrawal of care, the BIS value abruptly fell to less than 4 (point 4) and, simultaneously, heart rate decreased from 108 bpm to 0, and blood pressure dropped from greater than 100 Hg to less than 40 Hg. The patient was pronounced dead 32 minutes after the withdrawal of life support (point 5). Adapted from Auyong DB, et al. Processed Electroencephalogram During Donation After Cardiac Death [100].

occurred when the mind awoke and disengaged from the brain. During the disengagement process, the mind, as previously discussed, would theoretically have been able to influence the brain until the associated magnetic fields had, along with the mind, passed outside the sphere of influence in accordance with Coulomb's Law. The idea that mentally-induced magnetic fields can influence brain function, even from outside the fully intact skull, has been demonstrated by Grau et al.[29], who found that the magnetic fields that were induced by the thoughts of one person could be communicated to another person without the aid of somatic sensory organs.

Discussion

The well-documented observance of end-of-life electrical surges has added to the already heated debate about how to interpret NDEs, potentially providing a new line of support for a brain-based explanation for these extraordinary phenomena. Some clinicians and researchers argue that NDEs can be explained by the wave of death. Others say that NDEs are not necessarily related to this activity, pointing out that some NDErs have had verifiable experiences that were not necessarily linked to a specific time period post cardiac arrest[30], while others denied having had an NDE at all[30,31].

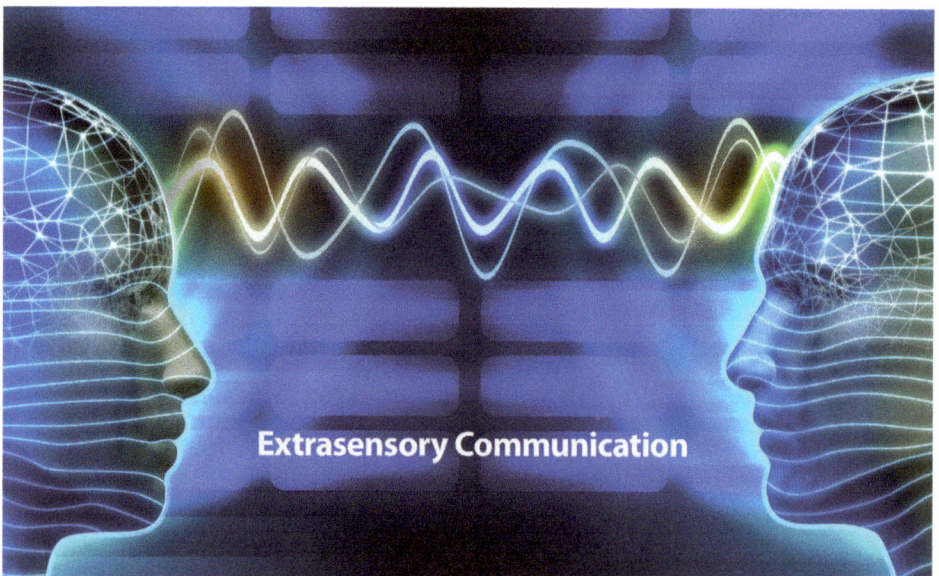

Extrasensory Communication

This analysis mitigates both sides of the argument with a new synthesis. It posits that the mind is an entity distinct from the brain yet dependent on it until it disengages from the brain at the time of death. This view allows for an anatomically and psychophysiologically-specific understanding of the seemingly conflictual data on end-of-life EEG activity. From the perspective of the mind-brain duality of the cognitive-emotional system, the mind drives neurological activity, and neurological activity drives mental activity. When this process is interrupted, either by a willful decision of the individual (the mind) or by a failure of the brain to dialogue with the mind, the mind falls asleep. This idea is supported by the observation that deep sleep, which under normal circumstances is initiated by the mind, is associated with a slowing of the EEG that is virtually indistinguishable from that seen in the comatose state[18].

In NDEs the mind seemingly awakens from this sleep. This is suggested by the close temporal relationship between the NDE, which by definition occurs during the transition from life to death, and the spike in synchronized brainwave activity that suddenly arises out of a flat EEG immediately prior to death. Yet despite this mental awakening, the body may remain clinically dead. This, taken together with reports that the duration of verifiable NDEs sometimes exceeds the duration of end-of-life electrical surges[30], implies that the mind must be separating from the brain and moving away from it during an NDE. This idea is consistent with the accounts of many NDErs, who say that they viewed their body from a distance, such as from the ceiling or the corner of the room. Additional support for the idea that the mind is separating from the brain during an NDE comes from a description that is common among NDEers; namely, that they experienced a heightened awareness and an expansion of their senses despite the fact that their brainwave activity was markedly diminished or even flatline leading up to and likely including much of the NDE. Among these are verifiable reports of blind persons being able to see and deaf persons being able to hear during the NDE *(YouTube: Vicki Noratuk NDE Vicki Noratuk NDE plus Radio Interview. BLIND person NDE, accessed 4/12/19, Kevin Williams NDE) (People Born Blind Can See During a Near-Death Experience. Accessed 5/16/18)*. The only conceivable explanation for these phenomena is that the mind is separating from the brain and reawakening outside the physical body. In theory, the associated mental and emotional activity could, during the transition process, drive a resurgence of brainwave activity just as occurs during the transition from deep sleep to rapid-eye-movement sleep and normal awakening from sleep. Though most NDErs say that they moved away from their bodies during the experience, the initial phase of the experience could still position the mind in close enough proximity to the brain to allow it to influence neuronal activity, especially because the experiences are so intensely vivid and emotionally captivating. This could explain why the spike in brainwave activity that has been observed immediately antecedent to the time of death is highly synchronized though brief. Note, however, that this phenomenon would not necessarily prevent the mind from returning to the body and regaining corporeal consciousness.

Based on this analysis, one could indeed say that NDEs are related to the surge of neurological activity that has been observed moments before death. However, I argue that it is not the surge that drives the NDE but the NDE that drives the surge. What may be happening is that the liberated mind is reawakening to life outside the physical body and that that awareness drives a surge of neurological activity that would be expected to approach, or perhaps due to the exhilaration of the experience, exceed that of corporeal conscious. That the mind can power the brain while simultaneously passing away from it is corroborated by the kinds of things that have been observed in dying patients as they pass from this life. Some experience heavenly visions; others become visibly agitated; and still others, though being severely obtunded, briefly become physically animated as they pass away[16,17]. Notably, some of those who display this last burst of physical vitality demonstrate knowledge and abilities that they did not have until they began to separate from their bodies, such as deaf persons being able to hear, blind persons being able to see, and cognitively impaired persons being able to recognize their loved ones again *(YouTube: What Really Happens When You Die | End-of-life-phenomena · At Home with Peter Fenwick)*. From this perspective, the most likely reason that most patients who have been successfully resuscitated do not report having had an NDE is that their minds did not detach from their bodies enough to wake up and have an NDE. In contrast, every laboratory rat that died in the Rijn[1] and Borjigin[2,28] studies would have left their bodies, thus explaining why every one of them expressed a death wave. These observations suggest the need to consider redefining death as a separation of the mind or, more accurately speaking, the spirit, from the physical body.

Curiously, however, not all human beings express an identifiable death wave immediately antecedent to the time that they are pronounced dead. According to the Chawla group, only about half of the patients who had EEG monitoring as they expired in the intensive care unit displayed end-of-life electrical surges[3]. One possible explanation is that a person could have left his or her body just prior to, or in the process of, lapsing into a coma and before any EEG monitoring had begun. Another possibility is that the same neurological abnormalities that interrupted the dialogue between the mind and the brain, thus leading to a comatose state, could have prevented the mind from effectively reactivating the brain when it began to separate from it. Yet another possibility is that such patients, having been pronounced clinically dead, had their monitoring equipment removed before their spirits actually left their bodies. It is also possible that they failed to separate from their bodies before their brains lost the capacity to generate neurological signals. What adds weight to this last possibility is that most patients who regain consciousness after being pronounced clinically dead do not report having had an NDE. These patients presumably remained asleep (and in their physical bodies) until the moment that they regained consciousness; hence the lack of an NDE.

Conclusion

The discovery of end-of-life electrical surges together with the growing number of verifiable NDEs strongly invokes the possibility that the mind is an entity distinct from the brain as has been proposed by some of the world's greatest scientists, philosophers, and thinkers. What the evidence related to end-of-life EEG activity suggests is that the mind, while asleep in the corporeal state, begins to separate from the brain and, in the process, suddenly awakens and stimulates a surge of neurological activity that corresponds to what it sees, thinks, and feels prior to passing outside the sphere in which its cognitive-emotional processes are able to influence the electrical activity of the brain. To my knowledge, this is the first anatomically, psychophysiologically, and electromagnetically-based explanation that links end-of-life EEG activity to near-death experiences without discounting the perceived extracorporeal nature of those experiences.

This theoretical formulation raises important questions about the criteria that are used to make a determination of death. While death has traditionally been thought of as a global shut-down of biological processes, the indicators that are used to make a determination of death are the same as those that are used to ensure that a patient under general anesthesia is adequately anesthetized. Clinical and electrophysiological indicators such as a loss of responsiveness to nociceptive stimuli, a loss of brainstem reflexes, and a pronounced slowing of the EEG occur in both the anesthetized and near-death states[18]. This again suggests that the transition from life to death involves something more than just a shut-down of bodily functions. That other something is also reversible, an observation that again points to the idea that death involves a separation of the energetic essence of a human being from the physical essence—the spirit from the body.

What is perhaps most reassuring is that any patient who meets established criteria for clinical death is either deeply asleep within the body or has passed away from the body, both of which minimize the chances of experiencing any pain or discomfort. Notwithstanding, the growing number of patients who are returning from the other side (thanks to medical advances in life support) argues strongly for the need to delay a determination of death for at least twenty minutes beyond the time that the patient meets clinical criteria for death. This would allow for the possibility that, until the time that the anoxic damage to the brain has become irreversible, the person who has left the body could still return to it and regain corporeal consciousness.

+ + +

References

1. van Rijn CM, Krijnen H, Menting-Hermeling S, Coenen AML. (2011). Decapitation in rats: Latency to unconsciousness and the 'wave of death.' PLoS ONE 6(1):e16514.

2. Borjigin J, Lee U, Liu T, Pal D, Huff S, Klarr D, Sloboda J, Hernandez J, Wang MM, Mashour GA. (2013). Surge of neurophysiological coherence and connectivity in the dying brain. Proceedings of the National Academy of Sciences. 110(35):14432-14437.

3. Chawla L, Seneff MG. (2013). End of life electrical surges. Proceedings of the National Academy of Sciences. 110(44)E4123.

4. Auyong DB, Klein SM, Gan TJ, Roche, AM, Olson DW, Habib AS. (2010). Processed electroencephalogram during donation after cardiac death. Anesthesia & Analgesia. 110(5):1428-1432.

5. Dreier JP, Major S, Foreman B, Winkler MKL, Kang EJ, Milakara D, Lemale CL, DiNapoli V, Hinzman JM, Woitzik J, Andaluz N, Carlson A, Hartings JA. (2018). Terminal spreading depolarization and electrical silence in death of human cerebral cortex. Annals of Neurology 83(2).

6. Zandt B-J, ten Haken B, van Putten MJAM. (2001). Neural dynamics during anoxia and the "wave of death." PLoS One. 6(7)e22127.

7. Norton L, Gibson RM, Gofton T, Benson C. (2017). Electroencephalographic Recordings During Withdrawal of Life-Sustaining Therapy Until 30 Minutes After Declaration of Death. Canadian Journal of Neurological Sciences 44(2):139-145.

8. Salman E. Qasim, Jonathan Miller, Cory S. Inman, Robert E. Gross, Jon T. Willie, Bradley Lega, Jui-Jui Lin, Ashwini Sharan, Chengyuan Wu, Michael R. Sperling, Sameer A. Sheth, Guy M. McKhann, Elliot H. Smith, Catherine Schevon, Joel M. Stein, Joshua Jacobs. Memory retrieval modulates spatial tuning of single neurons in the human entorhinal cortex. Nature Neuroscience. 2019; DOI: 10.1038/s41593-019-0523-z.

9. Wang S, Tudusciuc O, Mamelak AN, Ross IB, Adolphs R, Rutishauser U. (2014). Neurons in the human amygdala selective for perceived emotion. Proceedings of the National Academy of Sciences 111(30):E3110-E3119.

10. Jimenez JC, Su K, Goldberg AR, Luna VM, Biane JS, Ordek G, Zhou P, Ong SK, Wright MA, Zweifel L, Paninski L, Hen R, Kheirbek MA. (2018). Anxiety Cells in a hippocampal–hypothalamic circuit. Neuron. 97(3):670–683.e6.

11. Wang S, Yu R, Tyszka JM, Zhen S, Kovach C, Sun S, Huang Y, Hurlemann R, Ross IB, Chung JM, Mamelak AN, Adolphs R, Rutishauser U. (2017). The human amygdala parametrically encodes the intensity of specific facial emotions and their categorical ambiguity. Nature Communications. 8:14821.

12. Xu Y, Jia Y, Ma J, Hayat T, Alsaedi A. (2018). Collective responses in electrical activities of neurons under field coupling. https://doi.org/10.1038/s41598-018-19858-1.

13. Trimble M.R. (1989). The Prefrontal Cortex: Anatomy, Physiology and Neuropsychology of the Frontal Lobe. British Journal of Psychiatry.

14. Braun AR, Balkin TJ, Wesenten NJ, Carson RE, Varga M, Baldwin P, Selbie S, Belenky G, Herscovitch P. (1997). Regional cerebral blood flow throughout the sleep-wake cycle. An H2(15)O PET study. Brain. 120(7):1173–1197.

15. Solms M. (2014). The Neuropsychology of Dreams: A Clinico-anatomical Study (1 ed.). Psychology Press. ISBN: 978-1315806440.

16. Moody RA. (1975). Life after life. Mockingbird Books.

17. Fenwick P, Fenwick E. (2008). The art of dying. Continuum Books, New York, NY.

18. Brown EN, Lydic R, Schiff ND. (2010). General Anesthesia, Sleep, and Coma. New England Journal of Medicine. 263(27):2638-2650.

19. Lemmi H, Hubbert, CH, Faris, AA. (1973). The electroencephalogram after resuscitation of cardiocirculatory arrest. Journal of Neurology, Neurosurgery, and Psychiatry 36:997-1002.

20. Westhall E. (2016). Electroencephalography for neurological prognostication after cardiac arrest. Research output: Doctoral Thesis (compilation) Department of Clinical Sciences, Division of Clinical Neurophysiology, Lund University.

21. Posner JB, Plum F. (2007). Contemporary neurology series. 4. Oxford University Press; Oxford; New York. Plum and Posner's diagnosis of stupor and coma; p. xiv.p. 401.

22. Gottschalk A, Van Aken H, Zenz M, Standl T. (2011). Is anesthesia dangerous? Deutsches Arzteblatt International. 108(27):469-474.

23. Plaschke K, Boeckler D, Schumacher H, Martin E, Bardenheuer HJ. (2006). Adenosine-induced cardiac arrest and EEG changes in patients with thoracic aorta endovascular repair. British Journal of Anaesthesia. 96(3):310–316.

24. Binder M. (2019). The multi-circuit neuronal hyperexcitability hypothesis of psychiatric disorders. American Journal of Clinical and Experimental Medicine. 7(1):12-30.

25. Grunze HCR. (2008). The effectiveness of anticonvulsants in psychiatric disorders. Dialogues in Clinical Neuroscience. 10(1):77-89.

26. Blom EH, Serlachius E, Chesney MA, Olsson EMG. (2014). Adolescent girls with emotional disorders have a lower end-tidal CO_2 and increased respiratory rate compared with healthy controls. Psychophysiology. 51(5):412–418.

27. Schneider M. (1961). Survival and revival of the brain in anoxia and ischemia. In: H Gestaut & JS Meyer (Eds.), Cerebral anoxia and the electroencephalogram (pp. 134-143). Thomas: Springfield, Illinois.

28. Borjigin J, Wang MM, Mashour GA. (2013). Reply to Greyson et al: Experimental evidence lays a foundation for a rational understanding of near-death experiences. Proceedings of the National Academy of Sciences. 110(47):E4406.

29. Grau C, Ginhoux R, Riera A, Nguyen TL, Chauvat H, Berg M, Amengual JL, Pascual-Leone A, Ruffini G. (2014). Conscious brain-to-brain communication in humans using non-Invasive technologies. PlosOne. https://doi.org/10.1371/journal.pone.0105225.

30. Greyson B, Kelly EF, Dunseath WJR. (2013). Surge of neurophysiological activity in the dying brain. Proceedings of the National Academy of Sciences. 110(47)E4405.

31. Holden JM. (2009). The Handbook of Near-Death Experiences: Thirty Years of Investigation. JM Holden, B Greyson & D James (Eds.), pp. 185–211. Praeger Books, Santa Barbara, California.

Other Books By This Author

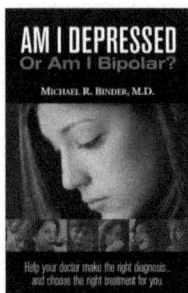

Am I Depressed Or Am I Bipolar?

This groundbreaking book will help you understand mood disorders from an anatomical, psychological, and spiritual perspective with an emphasis on making the distinction between classic depression and bipolar disorder. Drawing from years of clinical experience, research, and intensive study, board-certified psychiatrist Dr. Michael Binder unveils the anatomy of the mind and uses numerous case examples to familiarize you with the various forms that mood disorders can take. Throughout the book, he also discusses how they are properly diagnosed and treated.

Available at www.barnesandnoble.com and www.amazon.com

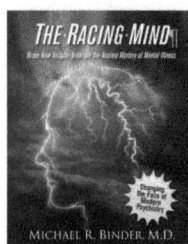

The Racing Mind

Persistent emotional distress is the most common ailment known to mankind. More than 80% of doctor visits are related to mental health issues, and psychiatric disorders are a leading cause of disability worldwide. Yet of all illnesses, these common disorders remain the most poorly understood. When we see people behaving out of the ordinary--becoming overly anxious, easily angered, highly moody, gravitating toward drugs, lapsing into depression--we naturally assume that their behavior is under voluntary control. Yet the little-known fact is that the brain, in distinction to the mind, is an emotionally-detached biological computer that is only partially under voluntary control.

This book is about the dynamic relationship between the mind and the brain and the way these two components of the cognitive-emotional system interact in sickness and in health. It is about how a subtle abnormality in brain function can leave one vulnerable to a spectrum of psychiatric symptoms from mild anxiety to florid psychosis and why persons with mental illness tend to die at an earlier age than the general population.

Available only through www.BinderFoundation.com

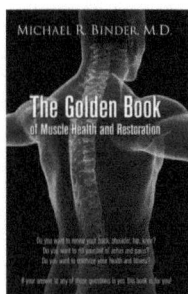

The Golden Book of Muscle Health and Restoration

The Golden Book is a revolutionary look at the hidden cause of chronic musculoskeletal pain and the only effective way to treat it.

Based on his own struggles with chronic pain and the brilliant work of Dr. Thomas Griner, Dr. Michael Binder addresses the little-known but extremely common problem of hypertonic muscle spasm. In this life-changing book, you will discover how hypertonic spasm develops, how it causes symptoms, and if you are already suffering from it's ill effects, what to do to get out of pain and stay out of pain without the need of drugs, injections, or surgery. We're talking about truths that are destined to revolutionize orthopedic medicine, physical rehabilitation, and the fitness world! So if you want to preserve the vitality of your muscles and get the most out of them; or, conversely, if you have ever thrown out your back, developed chronic pain in a joint, or experienced frightening symptoms like numbness, tingling, or pain down an arm or leg, this book is for you!

Available at www.barnesandnoble.com and www.amazon.com

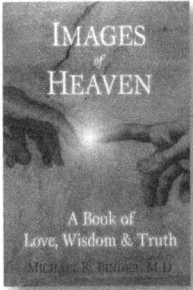

Images of Heaven: A Book of Love, Wisdom & Truth

This unique work is a study of the Holy Bible through the lens of science. Based on the most authentic complete Bible manuscripts in existence, Dr. Michael Binder combines his medical training and experience as a psychiatrist with the knowledge and insights of world-renown Bible scholar Dr. George M. Lamsa to help you understand the entire Bible, from the book of Genesis to the book of Revelation, in the language of our modern culture and times.

Images of Heaven is available only through The Binder Foundation. To learn more or to place an order, go to www.BinderFoundation.com.

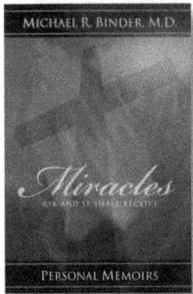

Miracles: Ask and Ye Shall Receive

Miracles is a book of personal memoirs that recounts the acts of God in the life of Dr. Michael Binder, a physician and scientist, who has witnessed the loving hand of God through faith time and again. Packed with more than one hundred miracles, this inspirational work describes the experiences of the doctor himself, which are presented with the historical accuracy and detail that one would expect from a clinical scientist. Those who believe in God will be strengthened by this book; those who are uncertain will be inspired; and those who do not believe will be challenged to take the leap of faith that opens the door to heaven on earth.

Available at www.barnesandnoble.com and www.amazon.com

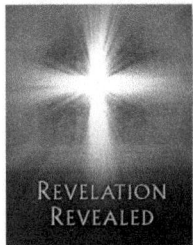

Revelation Revealed

For nearly two thousand years, the book of Revelation has been an enigma because it is so shrouded in Semitic idioms and cultural symbolism. In addition, the Revelation of Saint John, like all spiritual visions, transcends the limits of time, a characteristic that adds another layer of complexity that has led to uncertainty about such things as the timing of the rapture of the church and the thousand-year reign of Christ. Consequently, Bible scholars, theologians, and commentators have become caught in an unending debate about the interpretation of many passages of Saint John's vision. But God, in His grace, desires to reveal His glorious plans to his children; that is why He blessed Saint John with this prophesy of prophesies.

As the return of Jesus Christ draws near, the Lord has poured out a special blessing and opened up new insights into the message of this most dramatic, picturesque, and enigmatic book of the Bible. The cornerstone of these new insights is the recognition that Saint John's vision is actually a compilation of seven parallel visions that repeatedly describe the same sequence of events in much the same way that the first two chapters of Genesis provide two parallel accounts of the creation of the world, and the four Gospels provide four parallel accounts of the life, death, and resurrection of Jesus Christ.

When understood from this perspective, the sequence of events in the book of Revelation becomes crystal clear because the sequence is the same in all seven visions! Many other passages of the book of Revelation become clarified as well because properly decoding the sequence of events allows us to hone in on the time period of the events portrayed. Amen+

Available at www.barnesandnoble.com and www.amazon.com

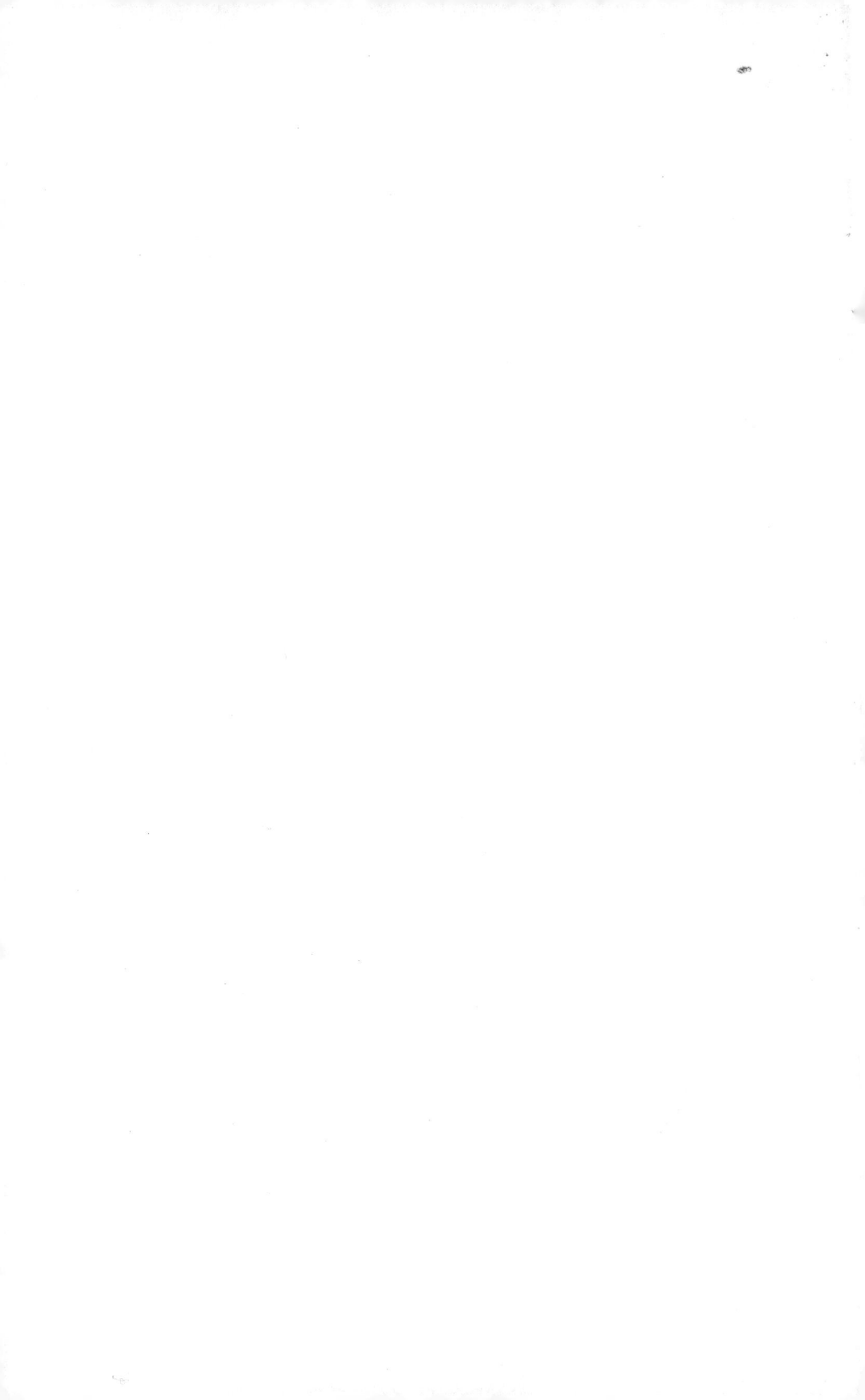